8 steps to a real-foods kitchen

Transform Your Kitchen
Transform Your Health

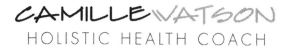

HOLISTIC HEALTH COACH

To contact the publisher, visit
www.createspace.com

To contact the author, visit
www.camillewatson.com

ISBN-13: 978-09961381-0-9
ISBN-10: 0996138102
E-book ISBN: 978-0-9961381-1-6

Cover and Text Design: Melissa Parker

Printed in the United States of America

Contents

*To my mom, who first taught me to cook
and enjoy real food.*

Acknowledgements

The dream of writing and publishing a book has been with me for most of my life. But dreaming of writing a book and actually writing the book are two very different activities. In the dream, it seems like a solitary venture. In reality, it takes an entire team of people. I want to thank all who encouraged me and worked beside me to make this a reality.

Thank you, editors Mariah Watson and Katy Ambrose, for dotting i's and crossing t's, and for ferreting out my unformed and unfinished thoughts. And thank you, Harrison Ambrose, for making me dig further to find the research to support my work. Melissa Parker, kudos to you for turning my fledgling ideas into a beautiful and professional graphic design. Joshua Rosenthal and Lindsay Smith, and the Institute for Integrative Nutrition® Launch Your Dream Book writing community provided instruction, support and camaraderie during this process. I could not have done it without all of you. Thanks to fellow author Rowen Marks for helping me keep on track as we worked out the kinks in our respective manuscripts. And to my husband, Brad Watson, who encourages me to go beyond myself: love you, sweetheart.

To my clients: this book is for you, my friends. You inspire me through your perseverance and the hard work you do to heal yourselves. Because of you, I have grown. Be nourished. Be well.

introduction

"You've been busy of late,
my friend."
Saruman[1]

YOU

These days you give and give, and take little time for yourself. You are juggling work, teacher meetings, trips to the doctor with your parents, and trying to have a good life with your family. You are hurtling forward in time at a breakneck pace. You look in the mirror and see signs of neglect: just like your yard when you are away, stuff sprouts. Other stuff breaks. But this is your health. You have seen enough to know that neglect will never serve you well.

At this point, you know a few things. Unlike your teenage son, who is sure he will live forever, you know you are not immortal. The writing is on the wall; if you stay on your current trajectory, you could end up with your parents' maladies. You are not willing to accept disease as your fate. You want your health back and you are committed. You will need to question the status quo—everything from what you eat to what you read in magazines to the prevailing popular wisdom for what constitutes healthy living. You want some answers, but you are just too busy to do all the research, to sift the facts from the fads. You could go it alone, but why not enlist some help? How great would it be if someone could package some good solid information all in one place—something to get you moving in the direction of better health?

ME

For me, health was always an elusive thing. As a kid, Sunday morning pancakes were a treat. The nausea afterwards was not. In high school I caught every cold and sinus infection going around, and had unexplained rashes. In college I was cold—very cold—always. Determined to live a healthier life, I majored in Nutrition. Soon after college I married the love of my life and entered graduate school in Computer Science. Again I fought colds, infections and the stress of all-night study sessions, heavy course loads and life as a graduate teaching assistant. Later I made beautiful babies and worked at a stressful job as a Data Analyst.

I applied what I had learned from my Nutrition studies about healthy eating. I ate lots of whole grains and legumes, made sure I cooked with "heart-healthy" oils, avoided most sweets, ate vegetables every day, and eschewed saturated fats and meats. In short, I applied the best of the prevailing nutritional wisdom of the day and my health deteriorated in the process.

THE MAZE

I have been blessed by those health challenges in my life because they forced me to keep a careful eye on nutritional developments in a field that is famously confusing. Over the years, new nutritional research has negated old beliefs over and again. Today a health "fact" may be considered indisputable, just to be replaced by a new health "fact" the next year. Some of these facts were never true, and some came from research that was later proven false. A couple of examples come to mind: back in the 1970s, "heart-healthy" polyunsaturated oils like corn, soybean and canola oil were being touted as the path to health. Today, we know that these inflammation-causing seed oils do not even make the list for healthy foods. During the same period, cereal was the only breakfast food that the health-savvy would consider. Now, newer research presents damning evidence of the disease potential of a heavily grain-based diet. In fact, during the early days of cigarette smoking, doctors were touting cigarettes as the path to health. The truth is, and your doctor will probably confirm this if you ask, nutrition classes comprise only a tiny percentage, if any, of a doctor's medical education.

One of the biggest problems with the myriads of nutritional information available is that some health "authorities" still believe, and quote, misinformation that is years out of date. And, sometimes sound nutritional advice is presented in a way that does not sound as sexy as the latest, greatest, sensationalized diet-with-a-big-name. No wonder this is all so confusing. It can be difficult to find your way in the maze.

Knowing how to feed your body for health does not have to be hard or overwhelming. As a matter of fact, when you eat as nature intended, it becomes simple. You eat beautiful, nourishing, satisfying foods. You heal.

A DELICIOUS JOURNEY

This book may contain ideas that sound radical to you. Hopefully it will change your relationship with food into one that is not only nourishing and sustaining, but also incredibly satisfying. Part recipe book, part instruction manual, it gives concrete information on transforming your kitchen and cooking practices so that the meals you create taste great and support your health. I give simple recipes to get you started. More importantly, I hope to give you the confidence you need to nurture and nourish your body with luscious, life-giving foods that you prepare.

I want you to know that vibrant health is possible. Through my relationship with real, whole foods, I now enjoy a greater level of health than ever before. And, as a Health Coach, I am able to teach my clients to overcome their health challenges by learning to prepare and savor delectable, soul-satisfying foods.

You are created to be healthy and whole. You are worthy of wellness. You can take back your health with nourishing foods. As you work through this book, pace yourself, go slowly, and enjoy the process of learning to cook real food. It is going to be a delicious journey.

step 1:
return to real foods

"'What is Real?' asked the rabbit one day . . ."
The Velveteen Rabbit[1]

My friend Harrison is a retired Biology professor and a really smart guy. He is having some trouble these days with diabetes, and he asked me what I thought he should do. "It's simple," I replied. "All you have to do is eat real food." I am not sure what I expected—maybe that he would have an enlightened look on his face as he exclaimed, "Oh, thank you for your sage and wise answer!" But instead, he looked at me, exasperated. "Cut the jargon." "Not jargon," I argued. "Real. Whole. Food. . . . Simple. Why is that jargon?" "Because," he said, "'Real Food' means something to you in your profession that I'm not familiar with. For instance, is sugar considered 'Real Food'? What about candy? Looks real to me."

WHAT IS REAL FOOD?

These days I am into "real" in a big way. I want deep and satisfying relationships with my family and friends. I want the clothing I wear to be of natural fibers that breathe. I want my hair to be the silver-shot blonde color that was hand-picked for me by Creation. I want the lotions and potions that touch my skin to be health-promoting—not full of untested chemicals. I want to breathe air in my home and community that is unpolluted. I want the water I drink and bathe in to be free of chemicals—clean and pure. And I want my food to be real and whole.

I know all of this is a lot to ask, but it should not be. Natural clothing just feels better, and it lets your body breathe. Deciding to return to my natural hair color is one of most empowering and radical things I have done lately. Not only am I no longer breathing chemicals from hair dye or letting them touch my skin, but it looks better. Skin absorbs about 60 percent of everything you put on it. Those chemicals on the skincare label that you cannot pronounce end up in the bloodstream. Clean water and clean air are getting more scarce than ever, but both are essential for good health.

I do not want to sound like everything has to be the same as it was a hundred years ago—our quality of life has changed in many ways for the better since then. But a couple of generations ago, people could take for granted that most food was good and nourishing. Large factory farms, agribusinesses, and processed foods have changed the nutritional landscape considerably in the time since then. These days, the word "real" requires some explanation. This, for me, is what real food looks like:

Real food appears very close to the way it does in nature. It is not highly processed or refined. It does not have a label, or if it does, the label is short and you can identify all the ingredients as food. It is found around the edges of the store in the produce, meat, and dairy sections (and some frozen food). Real food does not make health claims, or advertise with words like "New! Improved! Heart-Healthy!" It has not been changed in a lab or amped up with flavor enhancers, preservatives, or other chemicals. The very best real food is organic, in season, and locally grown. It is healing, sustaining and delicious.

When I was a kid, almost every Sunday my relatives would gather at my grandparents' home after church for a meal. On a regular Sunday there could be fifteen of us. On special occasions the ranks swelled to thirty or more. Because we were a traditional Southern family, the men would gather in the living room while the women put the final touches on the meal. Tables were set in the kitchen and dining room with fine china and everyday dishes. Granny would be at the stove, folding the final slab of butter into her nearly-famous fried corn. Grandaddy would be carving the roast or turkey he had put on to cook at 6:00 that morning.

Great bowls of new peas and salad greens would show up at spring dinners. Summer saw a proliferation of homegrown vine-ripe tomatoes, cucumbers, squash, eggplants and string beans. In autumn, turnips and turnip greens shared counter space with fried apples, "shelly" beans and mashed potatoes, rich and creamy with milk and butter. In winter, we would eat from the cellar—onions, sweet potatoes, home canned tomatoes and green beans, seasoned with traditionally cured country ham.

Those Sunday dinners not only provided me with great memories, but they sustained me in so many other ways. The food was whole and organic because in those days, most food was organic. Many of the vegetables were seasonal and locally raised by Grandaddy. He usually knew the farmer who raised the roast or turkey. Very little of the food was prepackaged unless it was canned by my grandparents. There was great color and variety in the meal—a feast for the senses. From a nutritional viewpoint, the color and variety provided a cornucopia of nutrients. The meal was deeply nourishing. And it was blessed and joyful, served with love and eaten with laughter. It sustained me and solidified my place in that big, noisy Southern family.

While these things are wonderful, you do not necessarily need grandparents, a big family, and your own garden to eat real food.

Here is another example, and one of my favorite quick and easy foods: a bowl of quinoa, slathered with the best olive oil you can find, and topped with sea salt. Add to this a green salad topped with an egg, and you have an fast breakfast, easy lunch or light dinner. Simple. Nourishing. Delicious. A feast in miniature.

DRIVE-THROUGH NATION

There are compelling reasons to change our eating habits. Americans today are eating at fast food restaurants more than ever. It is showing up on our waistlines and making us sick. Obesity is at an all-time high in this country, as well as inflammatory diseases like heart disease, diabetes, and cancer. The food we eat has fundamentally changed, and not for the better.

You know that fast food is bad for you. So why do you find yourself, a perfectly intelligent person with the best of intentions about your health, in the drive-through line? It goes something like this:

Monday morning has arrived. Your alarm was still set for Sunday, and did not go off until 7:00. That leaves you 45 minutes to get your kids to school and get yourself ready for work and out the door. You have just stepped out of the shower and are fishing for a towel and you remember they are all in the dryer, still wet. Your teenage son yells through the bathroom door that he has a report due this morning. He needs you to proof-read it. No, it cannot wait; it was actually due Friday, and he will get a zero if he does not turn it in today. And it is fully one-fourth of his semester grade.

Finally, at 8:25 you race out the door, remembering that at the end of your 35 minute commute, you will be in front of a room full of people making a presentation. The presentation goes . . . OK . . . and then you have another round of meetings. Suddenly, it is 12:30, and you are shaking from hunger. You have only had coffee and maybe a bagel this morning. And you have to be in the VP's office at 1:00 for yet another meeting. So, you find yourself in the drive-through, starving and completely out of willpower. You order the double steak-burger and fries combo (on sale for a dollar off today) and top it off with this-month's-special piña colada shake because, after all, you do need some calcium. You uneasily remember your triglycerides score from the last time you went to the doctor and tell yourself you will do better tomorrow. The meal tastes great—they always do because of the added chemical flavor enhancers—but leaves you feeling overly full, lethargic, headachy, and frustrated by thwarted goals and resolutions.

A change in your eating habits can make a profound difference in your health in a short period of time. Morgan Spurlock found this out in 2004 when he embarked on a 30 day diet of only McDonald's® food and documented his experience in the movie **Supersize Me**.[2] At the beginning of the 30 days, he met with three different doctors for a physical. All doctors found him to be in excellent health. None were worried about his little experiment. One thought his cholesterol level might go up a bit, but other than that, he was young and healthy and there was nothing to be concerned about.

Toward the end of the 30 days, his doctors were begging him to quit, and imploring him to go to the emergency room immediately if he felt any shortness of breath or chest pains. They were afraid he would not live to see the end of the experiment.

WHAT REAL FOOD CAN DO FOR YOU

What is the big deal about inflammation? Inflammation is a link in many major diseases including heart disease, cancer, Alzheimer's, arthritis, multiple sclerosis, Parkinson's disease, osteoporosis, diabetes, obesity, allergies (including asthma and food intolerances), chronic fatigue syndrome, fibromyalgia and many other pain disorders. Many of the highly processed foods sitting on grocery store shelves today can increase the inflammation in your body.

Too much information? Let me tell you, instead, what it feels like to eat real food. You sleep better. You have more energy and focus. Your blood-sugar stays put, so you do not feel the wild hunger strikes when it is way too early for lunch. Your immune system is stronger so you get sick less often. When you do get sick, your body can fight it better. You heal more quickly. Your joints quit hurting so much. And when you go to the doctor, you get good news, not bad. Your triglycerides are down. Your weight is closer to ideal. You can see your toes and touch them. You feel like walking or dancing or biking, or whatever body movement appeals to you.

I hear arguments against eating well. Here are a few of my favorites:

"I eat pretty well already. I don't think it's a big deal to eat processed food." None of us want to be fanatical about eating; to be perfect all the time is impossible and unsustainable. But before you decide that you are eating pretty well, first learn what that means in terms of the best information about nutrition, and take a look at your health. If your health needs to improve, you might want to consider working on your food and lifestyle first before you turn to prescriptions or over-the-counter quick fixes. May I suggest the 80/20 rule? Eat well 80 percent of the time, and relax a bit the other 20 percent. But if we strive for 80/20, we will actually come in at about 60/40. So, as Mark Sisson, author of **The Primal Blueprint** says, if your intentions for excellent eating are at 90 to 100 percent, you will reach your 80/20 goal.[3]

"But it tastes so bland." Processed foods contain hefty doses of flavor enhancers such as monosodium glutamate (MSG). MSG is an excitotoxin, which means that it has the ability to rev up your taste buds. What happens immediately is that you think what you are eating tastes amazing. Over the long term, you become addicted to foods containing these excitotoxins, and everything else tastes flavorless. When you decide to quit MSG and other excitotoxins, it may take a week or two for your amped up taste buds to calm down. Then you can begin to appreciate the incredible flavor of real food. On the other hand, one of the marks of really delicious food is that it is well-seasoned. So, season your food—I will show you how!

"I don't want to deprive myself." Neither do I. I often hear people say they want to eat better, but they are not excited about changing their eating habits. It is a process that takes time and a willingness to change. Know that once you get used to eating real food, you will prefer it, and will feel deprived if you do not get it. With real food, you can eat some of the best food on the planet. And you can have some sweets. Sweets were not a problem in the past because people ate them as an occasional treat, not as an every meal requirement. And, sweets of earlier generations tended to be made from more wholesome ingredients.

"I can't afford to eat all that expensive food." Eating healthy foods cost about $1.50 more per day per person than eating unhealthy foods, according to research from the Harvard School of Public Health. Researchers found that diets rich in fruits, vegetables, fish and nuts cost slightly more than unhealthy diets such as those rich in refined grains and processed foods. So, on average, a year's worth of the most healthy foods cost about $550 more per year per person than the least healthy ones.[4] Ask yourself how much your health is worth to you. Is it worth $1.50 a day to change your trajectory so that you are not courting major diseases? It is quite possible that you may save that much in medical expenses and lost work in the short term. And in the long term, you will reap real savings because you will be healthier. Michael Pollen sums it up best: "Although 'real' food is often more expensive . . . you either pay for real food now—or pay the doctor later. In 1960, 17.5 percent of our national income was spent on food, and only 5.2 percent on healthcare. . . Today, 9.7 percent of our income is spent on food and a whopping 16 percent on healthcare. The less we spend on food, the more we spend on healthcare."[5]

"I don't have time to cook everything from scratch." You may think that cooking real food requires hours of sweating in the kitchen. If you are used to popping something instant in the microwave or stopping at the drive-through on the way home, then yes, you will be spending more time in the kitchen. Cooking whole foods takes a different mindset. But it does not have to be difficult. A lot of the time, it is a matter of planning ahead. Many simple whole foods do not take much longer to prepare than their fast-food counterparts. And, cooking at the end of the day can be a way to unwind and spend time with your family. Good conversation and delicious smells will make you want to cook more often. I will show you ways to maximize taste while you minimize your time in the kitchen.

I challenge you to commit to your own health and longevity by committing to real food. Refuse to eat the over-processed, flavorless and excitotoxin-enhanced food-like substances that do nothing to sustain your body. Eat food that is fresh and life sustaining. Eat food with soul.

HOW TO BEGIN:

Easy changes you can make now:

- ✔ Read through this book, just to get a feel for the journey.

- ✔ Grab a piece of fruit for a snack instead of a cookie.

- ✔ Shop for lunch at a grocery store instead of a fast food restaurant.

- ✔ Become a master at creating inspired green salads. Eat a salad every day.

- ✔ Find the local food cooperative or farmer's market in your area.

Bigger changes to incorporate slowly over time:

- ✔ Commit to making changes over time. Work through this book slowly so that you can enjoy the process without feeling overwhelmed. Each week, replace one or two not-so-good-for-you foods with foods that are delicious and life-sustaining.

- ✔ Find a healthier alternative that is similar to your favorite junk food to replace it.

- ✔ Stop eating food in packages, or choose packages with a few wholesome ingredients.

- ✔ Become a label reader. Look for labels with few ingredients and make sure each ingredient is a whole food.

- ✔ Shop at the edges of the store in the produce, meat and dairy sections.

- ✔ Shop at your local food cooperative on a regular basis.

- ✔ Learn to love to cook. Start easy with some of the simple recipes in this book.

- ✔ Use cooking as a way to unwind and connect with your family.

step 2:
devise a (grocery) market strategy

"The only real stumbling block is fear of failure. In cooking you've got to have a what-the-hell attitude."

Julia Child

It is 6:00 p.m. and you just got home from work. You are looking in the fridge, and waiting for inspiration to strike (or for dinner to materialize). The freezer compartment is not offering any clues either. It seems pretty empty, except for some frozen lumps of . . . something. Before you decide to throw in the towel and forget about cooking altogether, you may just need a strategy for making dinner happen.

What would this strategy consist of? First, you need a plan, specifically a menu plan. This can be as simple as a short list of foods you like to eat at this particular time of the year. Then, you need a way of translating that plan into action. You need to know how to navigate the grocery store, discover the best foods and bring them home.

Almost every Friday morning when I was young, my mom and aunt would pile all of us cousins into the family car and head for the grocery store. Mom and Aunt Virginia would shop for our weekly groceries while we kids would try, and not very hard, to stay out of trouble. Uncle Earl, who worked at the store, would ring up our groceries. Afterwards, we could have a hamburger at

Krystal® for lunch if we had behaved ourselves. We did not often get hamburgers.

Interestingly, Friday morning was the only time we went to the store. There was no standing in line at 9:30 on a weeknight for forgotten ingredients, or stopping on the way home. Mom planned out her week, shopped once, and was done. The roast chicken we had on Monday evening became the chicken pot pie served on Wednesday. While the "Mrs. Cleaver-like" life is not the norm today, having a plan can still save a lot of time and money.

STRATEGIC PLANNING

I always hated menu planning. It seemed hard and stuffy, and looked like it would be a lot of work to cook everything on the menu. Oh, I would try to do a menu plan (after all, I am a foodie). I would pull out my recipe books and make an elaborate plan of all the recipes I wanted to cook. At first I would feel inspired. But as the week wore on, I never felt ambitious enough to cook all of the food on the menu. At some point I came to the realization that I was doing it all wrong. Rather than perusing cookbooks and trying to plan meals straight out of Betty Crocker®, it helps to look at a menu as a simple plan of action. The truth is that you can save a lot of time and money with a simple menu. Why time? Because you spend less time in the grocery store when you can purchase food for several meals at once. And money? Planning your menus helps you to cut down on unneeded purchases. I never leave the grocery store with only what I went in there for unless I have a plan. The less I plan, the more I spend.

The trick in planning a menu is to write down what you really think you will cook, not some grand idea of what you would cook in a perfect world. And while you are converting to a Real-Foods Kitchen, this is a good opportunity to include some real foods—broccoli that can be tossed in a saucepan to steam for a few minutes and then topped with olive oil and sea salt, a head of lettuce for a salad, or some Sock-Eye Salmon to be run under the broiler with dill weed, olive oil and sea salt. Here is how you do it: Jot down five easy main dishes that you might like this time of year. Next to each main dish, write in a green vegetable or salad to accompany it. Add a second vegetable in a different color or add a grain. Sometimes one-pot meals can serve as main dish and vegetable. Choose foods or recipes that are in keeping with the amount of time you like to spend in the kitchen. If one of the three menu items is a recipe with several ingredients, keep the other two simple.

A MASTER MENU

Here are some examples of simple meals. Leaf forward to the back of this book for the recipes.

- Salad Niçoise

- Grilled burgers with mushrooms and salad toppings, quinoa tabbouleh

- Quick spaghetti sauce with spaghetti squash noodles and a green salad

- Bubbies® chicken, oven-roasted broccoli & cauliflower, sweet potato salad

- Mediterranean skillet with rice

If you really want to save time, transfer all the ingredients you will need for your five dinners to a master grocery list. Now save the menu and the grocery list. Next time you want to cook these foods, copy both and take them to the grocery. You really only need a few menus per season that you can rotate. Do it once, reuse it again and again. Understand that this does not make you a slave to these particular dishes. You may be inspired to cook something different. If so, just add the new ingredients to your grocery list. The sample menu above has dishes that I would cook in spring and summer (Salad Niçoise, grilled burgers with mushrooms) and dishes that I would tend to cook in cooler weather (Mediterranean skillet, spaghetti). I also have some recipes that I turn to year round, such as Bubbies® chicken.

Once you have your menus and ingredients, you can vary the days, or decide to go out for one of the evenings. Remember to chill or freeze ingredients so they will be fresh when you decide to cook.

On every menu, try to have at least one thing that you make once and use twice. Here are some examples:

- Serve a roasted chicken one night, make soup or chicken salad out of it for another dinner or for a portable lunch.

- Make a pot of quinoa and find several ways to use it during the week.

- Make a crock-pot full of soup and freeze for future dinners or for lunches.

Keep this process simple. If you include complications, you will find yourself dreading the process. The idea is to get in the kitchen and get cooking to have quick and nourishing meals at the ready.

If you would love to have help planning a marvelous menu for each week, search the web for "menu planning." Look for a website which plans healthy menus using real food. You do not need anyone telling you to open another box. The best services will also generate a grocery list for you to carry to the store. Here are some of my favorites:

PlanToEat.com™ allows you to use recipes from different sources in planning your menus, either from the web or from your own collected recipes. After entering your recipes, you can add them to a calendar and then generate a grocery list.

CookSmarts.com™ develops and provides four new healthy recipes a week, plus an archive of previous meals. You can choose from special dietary needs like gluten-free or low-carbohydrate. CookSmarts generates a grocery list.

EatThisMuch.com™ automatically creates meal plans and grocery lists that meet your diet goals. It can be personalized for your food preferences, budget and schedule.

ON THE HOME FRONT

If you were only going to go the store once a week (not saying that you are), you would need a place to put your food when you got home. So, before you leave for the grocery, take five minutes to clean the "science projects" out of your fridge. Science projects include all the things that used to be food, but that you will not be eating in the future. You do not have to clean the whole refrigerator at one time. Pick one shelf, take everything out, wipe it down, and return the items that are still fresh. Do not turn this into a multi-hour project, or you will never find the time to get to it.

RECONNAISSANCE MISSION

We are going on a field trip. In your hometown there are, in all likelihood, a variety of food stores. There are the quick markets, the traditional grocery stores, and probably at least a few natural grocery stores and specialty markets. It is worth your while to seek out new places to shop. Quick food stores generally have a limited selection of expensive pre-packaged goods, along with a few last-minute items like bread and milk—not the best venue for healthy foods. More and more, traditional stores are stocking organic and wholesome foods. Buying healthy foods at traditional grocery stores encourages them to carry a larger variety. Natural food stores often seem more expensive than traditional food stores because they carry more organic and specialty items that come with a larger price tag. But you will also find a much larger selection of bulk organic foods at a lower price in natural food stores than you will at a traditional grocery store. For example, the traditional grocery in my hometown carries tiny bags of quinoa at inflated prices because it is considered a specialty item. The natural food stores, however, carry the same item in bulk at a much lower price per ounce. Herbs and spices, when purchased in bulk at a natural foods store, are also significantly lower in cost. Shop natural food stores for items you may not be able to find at a traditional grocery stores. There is no reason to go to three different grocery stores in a week. However, as you shop from week to week, go to different stores to become familiar with their offerings as you pick up the items you need.

Sometimes it is worth a stop at a specialty food market to have access to food that is not available at regular grocery stores. I purchase grass-fed beef, pastured pork and free-range chickens from my local butcher. There I find delicious and healthy meats not available anywhere else in town.

Now you have arrived at the grocery store, list in hand. If you take a moment to look around the store, you will see that the real food is at the edges, and the boxes and food-like substances tend to be in the center aisles. This means that the edges of the store are where you will want to do the bulk of your shopping: produce, meats, dairy, and frozen food sections.

DECONSTRUCTING FOOD LABELS

The best natural foods have no ingredients label at all. For instance, when you purchase an apple, it has only one ingredient: apple. When you do purchase a food with an ingredients label, look for short ingredients lists that name real whole food ingredients. Here are some examples of packaged foods you might find:

- **Instant Pudding and Pie filling.** *Ingredients: Sugar, modified corn starch. Contains less than 2% of natural and artificial flavor, salt, disodium phosphate and tetrasodium pyrophosphate (for thickening), mono- and diglycerides (prevent foaming), artificial color, yellow 5, yellow 6, BHA (preservative).* What is wrong with this label? Sugar is the first ingredient. It contains artificial ingredients and chemical names as well as artificial colors and preservatives.

- **Stroganoff boxed meal, just add hamburger.** *Ingredients: Pasta (whole wheat flour), Corn Starch, Salt, Enriched Flour (wheat flour, niacin, iron, thiamin mononitrate, riboflavin, folic acid), Modified Whey, Whey, Natural Flavor, Sugar, Yeast Extract, Potassium Chloride, Maltodextrin, Citric Acid, Onion, Ricotta Cheese (whey, milk fat, lactic acid, salt), Partially Hydroginated Soybean Oil, Parsley Flakes, Lactic Acid, Color Added, Calcium Lactate, Spice, Silicon Dioxide (anti-caking agent).* What is wrong with this label? There is a long list of ingredients, most of which are not names of real food. (Have you ever craved a big serving of Yeast Extract or Calcium Lactate?) Notice that some of the "real food" ingredients like parsley flakes occur later in the list, and therefore in smaller quantities, than non-food substances like maltodextrin.

- **Potato chips.** *Ingredients: potatoes, salt, maltodextrin, modified corn starch, cottonseed oil.* These potato chips contain additional ingredients that have no place in a healthy snack. Most notable is the cottonseed oil. Cottonseed oil is a product of the garment industry and is not regulated for heavy pesticide use.

- **Potato chips.** *Ingredients: organic potatoes, avocado oil, sea salt.* Some might argue that potato chips have no place in a real-foods kitchen. But if you are going to eat potato chips as an occasional indulgence, this ingredients list reflects real whole foods. Avocado oil is especially good for cooking at high temperatures because it does not degrade in high heat. Whether or not you can bring these chips home is going to depend on your level of self-discipline.

- **Organic canned tomatoes.** *Ingredients: organic tomatoes, sea salt.* This has a short ingredients list and both ingredients belong in a whole foods diet. I use this item a lot. Grab some and throw them in your cart for spaghetti sauce and Mediterranean cooking.

- **Organic peanut butter.** *Ingredients: organic peanuts, sea salt.* Short list. Check. Real ingredients. Check.

USING COUPONS

In my Sunday paper there is always at least one insert that is full of grocery store coupons. I remember when I was growing up that my Mom would carefully clip and file all of the coupons in the Sunday paper that might help her save on our grocery bill. As a stay-at-home mom, she counted this as her contribution to our family's financial welfare, and was very serious about the amount she saved on our food bill. Even today, there are many people who rely on coupons, sometimes saving large portions off their food bill. The bad news is that many of these coupons are for higher priced and packaged food that may not benefit your health. Real foods usually do not come pre-packaged and are largely unadvertised. When was the last time you saw a coupon in your Sunday paper for fresh, organic carrots? The good news is that, since the best foods are not heavily advertised, you are not paying for an advertising budget. If you do find a coupon for something healthy that you would be purchasing anyway, by all means use it. Many natural grocery stores have their own coupons. Look for them at the front of the store or on the store's website or email list.

KNOW YOUR FARMER

A great tragedy here in America is that the small farmer is a dying breed. It is incredibly difficult for small farmers to compete price-wise with the large mega-farms that are producing cheap food. Many family farmers have turned to a new market: organically raised produce, and naturally pastured animal and dairy products. These farmers can be found in farmers markets; their brands can be found on labels in food cooperatives, and sometimes at farm-to-consumer stands or stores. I trust my farmers because I know them, and I have had the opportunity to visit their farms. I have looked them in the eye and asked if their food is organically raised and if they treat their livestock humanely. Yes, their foods are more expensive, but the quality is unsurpassed. Every time I shop, I am supporting a hard-working family and I get to be an agent for social change.

RESOURCES FOR REAL FOOD

- **Conventional Grocery Stores:** Regular grocery stores are carrying more and more organic produce and packaged goods. The organic produce may be side-by-side with the conventional, or it may be in its own section. Packaged organic goods at conventional stores are often found in their own section.

- **Natural Grocery Stores:** A new breed of stores, natural grocery stores emphasize healthy eating and bring a larger selection of organic, sustainably grown, fair trade foods. They are becoming easier to find, even in smaller locales. These stores sometimes are independent, but more likely have a corporate presence. Whole Foods®, Trader Joe's® and Earth Fare® are examples.

⚫ **Food Cooperatives:** A food coop is a grocery store that is owned by its members. The one in your area may be a small, quaint place, or it may be large and modern. The one in my hometown began over 30 years ago as a tiny storefront in an old building. It has now expanded and renovated, and it rivals the corporate natural food stores in the area. There, you are likely to find local foods and pastured meats and eggs. You will find Fair Trade items (meaning the workers were treated fairly and paid a living wage) and unusual foods. You can also find packaged goods where every ingredient on the label is a real food.

⚫ **Food Buying Groups:** There are companies who will bring the grocery store to your town. It works like this: A group of people band together to place a minimum order, and agree to be on hand when the order is delivered. At the appointed date and time, the semi-trailer truck arrives and disperses food that has been prepaid. There is usually a coordinator for this type of food buying group. Health venues (such as nutrition stores and yoga studios) and groups of families (such as churches) will often be aware of the food buying groups in your community.

⚫ **Farmers' Markets:** Every year during the darkest days of winter I begin to look forward to spring and the opening of our local farmers' market. It is a great way to shop for locally produced vegetables, fruits and meats, and to meet the farmers who grow your food. Here, you may also discover unique local crafts and artisans.

● **Farm-to-Table Stores and Stands:** Local fruit stands, complete with home-made cardboard signs abound in the summer. This is a great way to pick up local produce. There are also year-round stands and permanent farm-to-table stores for produce and meats.

● **Community Supported Agriculture, or CSAs:** When you become a member of a CSA, you purchase a share of vegetables from a local farmer. You agree to pay a set price all summer long and, in return, you get a weekly supply of fresh, and often organic, vegetables from your farmer. This helps farmers because the members share the financial risks involved in growing fresh produce. And it gives you access to farm-fresh produce at excellent prices.

step 3:
stock your
pantry

"Let thy kitchen be thy apothecary;
and let foods be thy medicine."

Hippocrates

You have made a list, gone to the store, and brought the food home. Now, where will you put it? After you have stored produce and cold goods, the rest belongs in your pantry. A pantry can be a separate closet in your kitchen, or it can be a hall closet near your kitchen, a cupboard or a piece of furniture. You can even use a couple of study boxes or a garage shelf if you do not have a pantry. Why have a pantry? You can save time, money and energy by having stored food. And you'll be better prepared for life's emergencies. Without a place to store staples, you will find yourself running to the store more often and buying foods you do not need.

JETTISON THE JUNK

One of most important steps in converting your kitchen into a haven for healthy foods is to get rid of foods that are detrimental to your health and to replace them with foods that nurture your health. You may be a thrifty person and want to use up what you have before replacing it, but often this is an invitation to put off the transition to healthy foods. Make a commitment to get these foods out of your house now, and begin today to create a healthy kitchen. How do you tell which foods should remain and which should leave your kitchen? Become a label reader. Here is a list of ingredients that should leave your home immediately:

High Fructose Corn Syrup (HFCS). While all sugar in excess can contribute to obesity and major diseases like cancer and heart disease, high fructose corn syrup comes with its own special set of problems. High fructose corn syrup is extracted from cornstalks using a series of chemical processes. The resulting substance is neither natural nor healthy. High fructose corn syrup is found in poor quality, nutritionally deficient foods. It is cheaper and sweeter than sugar, and is absorbed into the body more rapidly. It causes a buildup of fat in the liver and triggers unhealthy spikes in insulin. High fructose corn syrup does not belong in a healthy kitchen.

Refined Vegetable Oils. Back in the 1970s, polyunsaturated oils became the newest and hottest health savior. More recently, canola has been dubbed the darling of cooking oils. Since then, researchers have determined that these liquid canola, sunflower, safflower, corn and soy oils contain large amounts of omega-6 fatty acids which cause inflammation in the body. While our bodies do need small amounts of omega-6, consuming grain and seed oils gives us too much. Many of these oils are genetically modified, and contain pesticides and other toxins. Most are chemically extracted, which adds insult to the inflammation. Expeller pressed versions, those squeezed under pressure to extract the oils, are better than those produced by chemical extraction. But the resulting seed oils still contain excessive omega-6 fatty acids. These oils are widely used because they are cheap, but they are not health promoting.

If you find a packaged food containing cotton seed oil, put it back on the shelf and step away quickly. Cotton seed oil is especially problematic because the seeds come from the apparel industry. There are no upper limits on the amount of pesticides that can be used on this crop because it is intended for clothing, not food. According to the Pesticide Action Network, "Conventionally grown cotton uses more insecticides than any other single crop. Nearly $2.6 billion worth of pesticides are sprayed on cotton fields each year—accounting for more than 10% of total pesticide use and nearly 25% of insecticides use worldwide."[1] The oils in the seeds from apparel cotton are chemically extracted by the food industry. The resulting cotton seed oil is used in producing cheap food items.

Hydrogenated Oils and Trans Fats. Hydrogenation is a process by which liquid oils are made solid at room temperature by zapping them with high-pressure hydrogen. While some of these liquid oils may be healthy in their natural state, hydrogenation renders them unhealthy. Trans fats are produced by hydrogenation. Trans fats wreak havoc on our health by raising bad cholesterol levels, thickening the blood, and causing lesions on artery walls. Luckily, laws were enacted several years ago that limit the use of trans fats in foods. Unfortunately, labeling laws in the US allow small amounts of trans fats into packaged foods that are labeled with "No Trans Fat." Whether or not the label indicates trans fats, if the word "hydrogenated" is in the ingredients list, that food contains trans fats. Just say no to anything that is labeled "hydrogenated"—your heart will thank you.

Artificial Colorings. If you read through the fine print on the FDA's website,[2] you will find that seven artificial colors are allowed for use in food products. The list used to be longer. Some of these seven colorings have been banned in other countries. The European Union requires a warning label on foods containing artificial colorings, but the United States does not. Some of these colorings have been found to cause behavioral problems as well as tumors and birth defects in lab animals.[3] So what are they doing in our food? People are drawn to foods that look like they were just picked. A pickle that is enhanced with green food coloring looks more "natural" and more appealing than a pickle that has turned grey. Some of the foods we have grown up with, like flavored gelatin and children's cereals would be completely unappealing if the dyes and colorings were removed. Steer away from artificial colors in your cupboard. Instead eat from the cornucopia of beautiful colors in fresh vegetables. Certified organic foods contain no artificial colors.

Natural Flavors. It would be easy to tell you to avoid artificial flavors and only include natural ones in your food, but that would not tell the whole story. The FDA does not actually have a definition of "natural flavorings."[4] Any flavor not derived from a synthetic or artificial source can be deemed "natural." This gives the food industry carte blanche for all sorts of bizarre additives such as vanilla flavor made from cow manure.[5] Some "natural flavors" may be perfectly OK. The problem is that we do not know which ones. The best way to avoid artificial (and natural) food additives is to eat real, whole foods that come in the package nature provided for them.

Monosodium glutamate (MSG). MSG is a flavoring agent added to many processed foods. While it has little flavor itself, it causes food to taste delicious by exciting your taste buds. According to the book *Excitotoxins, The Taste That Kills*,[6] MSG can damage the brain and nervous system and plays a role in neurodegenerative diseases such as Alzheimer's disease. I am not interested in food additives which are described as toxins, so I choose not to have foods in my home that contain added MSG.

WHAT TO KEEP IN YOUR PANTRY

The short answer to what to keep in your pantry is that you should stock it full of healthy foods. Rather than give an exhaustive list, which would be cumbersome, expensive and confusing, I am going to give you the starting point: the items that I always keep in my pantry. From there, as you plan to cook new and healthy recipes, you can purchase ingredients for those recipes.

Bulk Items. Many natural foods stores sell items that can be purchased in bulk. These include nuts, fruits, granolas, grains, sugars, flours, herbs and spices. These items are found in covered bins. You scoop out the amount you want to purchase, write a stock number on the bag, and are charged by the pound. Items purchased in bulk are a better value than similar items that come pre-packaged. Less packaging is also more environmentally sound. These items in bulk bins are often quite fresh because many people purchase dry goods this way. In the beginning you will want to purchase just what you need for a new recipe. You can return and purchase extra once you know how often you will be using the food. I purchase many items this way, including quinoa, sea salt, herbs and nuts. Once you bring the bulk items home, make sure to store them properly so that they will remain airtight, away from sunlight and dry until use.

My favorite containers for storing goods in my pantry are inexpensive wide mouth quart and pint canning jars. With glass jars, you can easily see the contents. Because of the markings on the jar, you instantly know how much you have of an item. They keep dry goods fresh and prevent the spread of weevils and other critters. If you store dry goods in your pantry in plastic bags, these bugs can spread from food to food.

But why would you find a weevil in the first place? Many conventional dry goods are irradiated and contain pesticides and additives to prevent infestation. But the irradiation and pesticides are not good for your body. Think about this: do you want to eat something that a bug would turn its nose up at? Infestations are not a problem if you store your dry goods in glass jars. I always write the month and year of purchase on my dry goods jars. In general, plan to use herbs and spices and other dry goods within six months of their purchase for optimal flavor. Toss them if they have not been used in a year.

Grains. Confusion about grains abounds. The FDA, until recently, wanted us to eat twelve servings of grains a day. Now they advise at least three servings a day. Vegans and vegetarians extol grains as a way to get protein. The Paleo camp vilifies all grains. Grains do contain nutrients that are beneficial. But they also contain anti-nutrients called phytates, which bind other nutrients and carry them out of the body. Phytates are hard to digest. Large portions of grains can be harmful for digestive health, and they can cause your bathroom scales to tip in the wrong direction.

Wheat is of special concern. According to Dr. William Davis in his book ***Wheat Belly***,[7] the wheat found in items on grocery store shelves today bears little resemblance to the wheat found before the 1940s. At that time, wheat was hybridized to cause it to be shorter and stockier so that its stalk would not tear up when it passed through the combines. This "improved" wheat accounts for most of the wheat in the world today. It produces higher yields and contains more protein and gluten. This sounds good, but the modern, hybridized wheat was never tested on humans. It turns out that this wheat is harder to digest. This may be one of the reasons why we are hearing of so many people these days who have celiac disease and gluten intolerance. Whether or not wheat has a place in your kitchen depends on the stamina of your digestive system. If you are having any digestive difficulties, give this over-used grain a rest.

All this said, grains can be a part of a healthy diet. The best way to eat grains is to prepare them traditionally by soaking them first. Soaking grains in water overnight, and then discarding the water, neutralizes about 70 percent of the phytates. Add additional water or broth and cook well. The resulting grain is much easier to digest.

Rolled oats have a place in a real foods kitchen. They can be soaked overnight for a delicious breakfast porridge called Overnight Oatmeal, and can be added to baked recipes. Oats do not naturally contain gluten. However, most commercial oats are processed with the same equipment as wheat, and are therefore contaminated. Gluten-free oats are available for those with gluten sensitivities.

My favorite grain is quinoa (pronounced "keen-wah"). At any given time I usually have quinoa soaking or cooking in my kitchen. Other options include brown or white basmati and jasmine rice, amaranth, millet, teff and buckwheat. You can easily find these flavorful grains at a natural foods grocer.

Canned Goods. In late summer, when Grandaddy's garden was rich and ripe, I spent many a morning at my grandparents' house helping with canning. The dreaded job of washing the jars always fell to me because my hands were small enough to fit inside. We would can green beans, tomatoes, sauerkraut and pickles. The storage room in the cellar was filled to capacity with canned goods by the end of the growing season. Come winter, these beautiful and delicious jars of food would be served at Sunday feasts.

Home canning is enjoying a resurgence today. It can add dimension to a real foods kitchen. However, it is a hobby that requires time, commitment and equipment. Consequently, most of us turn to commercially canned goods. Vegetables and fruits lose some of their nutrients when canned, so in general, it is better to use fresh or frozen when possible.

There is a lot of controversy over the plastics used in the lining of cans. Plastics, in general, contain chemicals that are hormone disruptors. BPA is one of those chemicals. Some companies are removing the BPA from their can linings, but they are not necessarily disclosing the other chemicals in use in the linings of their cans. Your best bet is to minimize your use of canned goods, and use fresh and frozen foods. I purchase very few canned goods. When I do I look for BPA-free brands and stock my pantry with the following organic basics: tomatoes and tomato sauce, beans, pineapple, corn, pumpkin puree, olives and broths. As with other foods, choose canned goods with ingredients that are pronounceable, real foods.

Herbs and Spices. Every summer, my dad grew a garden. Now, this was no ordinary garden. It was the kind of garden you would see in a gardening magazine. Every plant was nurtured and coddled. The rows were straight, the tomatoes were perfect, and weeds were simply not allowed. One year I begged for a spot of soil and planted herbs in a corner of his garden fiefdom. He was not pleased that I was using precious space for my "weeds." So I made him a roast and new potatoes, seasoned with fresh rosemary. After that, his perfect gardens always included rosemary. He gave away cuttings to his friends, and extolled rosemary as if he were its original inventor. If you have a small patch of yard or a pot on a sunny window sill, grow yourself a small herb garden. Herbs are hearty and grow like weeds, so you cannot mess them up.

Herbs and spices add loads of flavor, but many people are hesitant to use them, thinking that there is a particular right or wrong way. Start out with a few basic herbs and spices and then begin experimenting. Buy your dried herbs and spices in small bulk quantities at natural food stores. This will yield a fresher, often organic product that costs a lot less than the little tins at a conventional grocery store. Spice mixes often contain fillers, preservatives and flavor enhancers (just read the label). It is better to mix your own.

Later you may want to invest in a mortar and pestle or use a re-purposed coffee grinder for the whole dried forms of herbs. Just as it is with coffee, grinding herbs as you use them releases even more flavor. But begin now with ground dried herbs; just measure and add to your food. What follows is a list of herbs and spices used in the recipes in this book; these are my favorites. Add a teaspoon or two to these to dishes and see if you like the result. Or add more to taste.

- Sea salt—a healthy alternative to regular table salt. Look for sea salt that has color: speckled Real Salt from the Redmond company, Himalayan pink sea salt or grey Celtic salt. The color in the salt is indicative of important trace minerals present. If sea salt appears pure white, it may have been bleached and stripped of its minerals. Add sea salt to your cooking instead of regular processed table salt. Regular salt has no minerals other than sodium chloride. When you crave salt, your body is actually craving minerals. If you use regular salt, you may continue to crave them because your body will not get the minerals it needs. Get your iodine by adding sea vegetables or a sprinkle of kelp to your food. Keep your refined table salt to throw on the front porch in an ice storm.

- Rosemary—Crumble dried rosemary in your hand or in a mortar and pestle, then add to green beans, pork, and beef dishes. Toss the twigs on your charcoal grill to infuse flavor into grilled steaks. If you are feeling adventurous, grow a rosemary bush for exceptional flavor.

- Thyme—Pronounced "time." Sprinkle fresh or dried thyme on your eggs, fish or pork chops. Add to soups and stews. Mix with other herbs for roasted herbed potatoes. Add to peas and carrots, or most anything that needs to rise above the everyday.

- Basil—Basil tastes like summer. Make pesto, add to Italian dishes or anything that calls for tomatoes. In August, slice tomatoes and mozzarella cheese and garnish with chopped fresh basil, then drizzle with balsamic vinegar for an impromptu Caprese salad. Add dried basil to soups in the winter.

- Oregano—Quintessential Italiana. In the winter, add dried oregano to great vats of spaghetti sauce that you can freeze. In the summer, stir-fry garlic in olive oil, add fresh red and yellow tomatoes, sea salt, pepper, basil and oregano for a memorable fresh spaghetti sauce. Add to your own version of Herbes de Provence, which is good on just about everything.

- Bay leaves—Add a leaf to anything soupy or saucy for added flavor. Try it in vegetable soup or spaghetti sauce. Remove the leaf before serving.

- Cinnamon—I love cinnamon in gluten-free muffins and sprinkled in my coffee. Cinnamon is sometimes used on meat dishes in Greek and Middle-Eastern cooking.

- Paprika—I keep both regular and smoked paprika on hand to add to roasted vegetables and to my soon-to-be famous Bubbies® Chicken recipe. I love the flavor and color it gives to chicken.

- Onion Powder and Garlic Powder—Keep these on hand for an extra dash of flavor.

Cooking Oils. Now that you have thrown away oils made from canola, safflower, sunflower, corn, soy, cottonseed and all hydrogenated oils, what do you replace them with?

- Olive oil—The flavor of high quality, extra-virgin olive oil is one of my great pleasures in cooking and eating. It is my favorite oil for salad dressings and drizzling on finished foods. It is high in inflammation-busting antioxidants called phenols and high in mono-saturated fatty acids which can help lower cholesterol and control insulin levels. Olive oil is best when it is never heated because it has a low smoke-point. Light olive oils have a higher smoke point, but are processed, sometimes at high temperatures. Once olive oil is heated it loses some of the qualities that make it exceptionally healthy. I do use olive oil sometimes for stir-frying vegetables just for the wonderful flavor.

- Coconut oil—A couple of decades ago people were sure coconut oil would kill you because it was always hydrogenated. More recently it has been vilified because it contains saturated fats. But suddenly, it has become the darling of health seekers everywhere, and for good reason. Coconut oil boasts a long list of health benefits. It has anti-viral, antibacterial, and anti-protozoa properties. It is easily digested, promotes heart health and promotes weight loss.[8] The coconut oil you find these days on the shelves of natural food stores is cold pressed and "extra-virgin," which retains the delicious flavor of the coconut. "Expeller pressed" can be used in cases where the coconut flavor is not desired. Coconut oil has a high smoke-point, so it is good for frying, baking and stir frying. In short, extra-virgin coconut oil is a super food, and a far cry from the old hydrogenated coconut oil.

- Avocado oil—Like olive oil, avocado oil is high in cholesterol-lowering monounsaturated fatty acids. But unlike olive oil, avocado oil has a high smoke-point. Avocado oil has a neutral flavor. Use this oil for frying and stir frying.

Packaged Foods. What packaged foods should you keep in a healthy pantry? The short answer is that you keep packages for which you can read and understand all the ingredients. Those ingredients should not include chemicals, preservatives, or colorants. The fewer the ingredients the better. For example, here are the ingredients of my favorite brand of cracker: *organic whole grain brown rice, organic whole grain quinoa, organic brown flax seeds, organic brown sesame seeds, filtered water, sea salt and organic wheat-free tamari (water, whole soybeans, salt, organic alcohol or organic vinegar).* Get in the habit of reading labels when you go to the grocery store. You will find companies you trust, and you can skip reading their labels on repeat purchases. Label reading becomes incredibly important if a member of your family has food sensitivities. Eventually label reading will become second nature, and you will know that the food in your pantry is wholesome.

CHECKLIST: A GOOD PANTRY

This chapter has a lot of information. But, after all, a good pantry is at the heart of a real-foods kitchen. Do not feel like you have to make all of these changes in a day. But do commit to making sure your pantry supports your move toward health with these steps:

- ✅ Jettison foods containing: high fructose corn syrup, seed oils, hydrogenated oil, artificial food coloring, artificial flavors and monosodium glutamate. Also get rid of products containing chemical names that do not sound like real foods.

- ✅ Purchase healthy foods in bulk when possible. Store in glass jars.

- ✅ Fill your pantry with organic grains including quinoa, oatmeal and rice. Resolve not to be dependent on wheat for your grains.

✔ Begin your foray into cooking with herbs and spices by adding the following dried herbs and spices: sea salt, rosemary, thyme, basil, oregano, bay leaves, cinnamon, and paprika. Toss the plain table salt.

✔ Purchase these oils to prepare healthy fare: avocado, olive, coconut.

✔ Toss packaged foods that have unreadable labels. Replace with healthier versions whose label contains only whole food ingredients.

step 4: get your fruits & veggies

"If you like to talk to tomatoes,
if a squash can make you smile,
if you like to waltz with potatoes
up an down the produce aisle . . ."

Theme song from Veggie Tales[1]

My sister-in-law once confided to me that she thought vegetables tasted boring. "How do you fix them?" I asked. "I boil them in water." "And?" I prompted. "Thats all. I just boil them until they are soft." "No sea salt? No herbs? No olive oil?" I asked, aghast. She shook her head. "I don't know what herbs to add."

If you open up any book on nutrition, it will tell you to eat a lot of fruits and vegetables, it will warn you darkly that most of us do not eat enough, and it will tell you to eat more than you are eating now— five servings a day! Seven servings a day! Yet I find that people get bored with fruits and vegetables, and do not know how to happily consume the required amount. The key to getting the nutrients you need is to eat enough of a variety of fruits and vegetables. The key to loving the flavor lies in choosing the freshest and best quality, and knowing how to prepare them.

EAT COLORFULLY

Imagine that you have two white plates in front of you. The plate on the left has a serving of fish and some brown rice on one side. The other side is filled with a big serving of steamed cauliflower. On the second plate there is an identical serving of fish and brown rice. But this time you have added some paprika and a slice of lemon to the fish. You chop some fresh parsley and scatter it over the fish and rice. The other side of the plate is filled with a fresh organic salad of spinach, grape tomatoes and purple onion slices with a citrus vinaigrette dressing. You roasted the cauliflower with broccoli, avocado oil, some sea salt and pepper added to that as well. Now, which plate would you prefer?

When you are striving for your servings of vegetables and fruits each day, it helps to dream in color. The more colorful the vegetables on your plate, the more variety of nutrients you are getting. The pigments in plants are powerful antioxidants. The red pigment in tomatoes is called lycopene. Green leafy vegetables get their color from chlorophyll. Carotene is found in carrots, oranges and squash. Anthocyanin gives blueberries their color. Antioxidants provide many health benefits because of their ability to neutralize free radicals in the body. Free radicals are produced as a normal process of metabolism and cause damage to your body.[2]

We could talk about serving sizes and number of servings, but an easier way to manage this is to look at your plate. Fill at least half of your plate with a variety of colorful fruit and non-starchy vegetables. Fill the remaining half with protein, whole grains, and starchy vegetables. The best way to ensure that you are getting all the nutrients that your body needs is to eat a cornucopia of colorful fruits and vegetables every day.

EAT SEASONALLY, EAT LOCALLY

These days you can get any fruit or vegetable you want at any time of the year. It was different not so long ago. There was a time when asparagus was only available in the spring, tomatoes were a summertime indulgence, and oranges were a treat reserved for the holiday season. You may think that only having some food available during certain times of the year is limiting, but is it really? Eating foods in season has many benefits, including better flavor, higher nutrition, lower cost and simply being in touch with the rhythm of the natural world. Meals are simplified by choosing foods in season. Freshly picked fruits and vegetables are a powerhouse of nutrients compared to plants that have been shipped half-way across the world. And there is nothing like the smell and taste of a tomato freshly plucked from the vine or chosen from a local farmer's stand in the heat of August.

Eating this way also offers the body unique seasonal benefits. Asparagus and dandelion greens are cleansing in the spring. Cucumbers and fresh salad greens are cooling in the summer. The vibrant pigments in tomatoes, watermelons and blueberries offer natural sun protection when eaten.[3] Root vegetables such as sweet potatoes are warming and grounding during the autumn. The vitamin C in citrus fruits boost the immune system in the winter.

Choosing local allows you to begin eating your produce soon after it is harvested. Fruits and vegetables begin losing nutrients as soon as they are picked. When they are shipped great distances, they must be harvested well before they are ripe in order to survive the journey. Later they are gassed with ethylene gas to ripen them. When they arrive in the store, the fruits and vegetables may look ripe, but do not have the flavor or nutrient profile of those that have been allowed to vine ripen. Many foods are irradiated as they are shipped as well. Shipping foods over distances has a substantial impact on pollution and greenhouse emissions. According to the National Resources Defense Council, "Imports by airplane have a substantial impact on global warming pollution. In 2005, the import of fruits, nuts, and vegetables into California by airplane released more than 70,000 tons of CO_2, which is equivalent to more than 12,000 cars on the road.[4]"

A final reason to seek out locally grown produce is the ability to get interesting and unusual produce, often heirloom varieties, in colors and flavors that you have never seen before.

HOW TO EAT VEGETABLES

Preparing fresh vegetables can seem intimidating. But it does not have to be. There are a few universal options for preparation that work for most all vegetables. I use these methods daily:

Eat them raw. Fresh raw vegetables are living foods and contain enzymes which are necessary for good digestion. Many vegetables need no preparation at all to taste delicious, especially when paired with healthy condiments. Try these ideas: baby carrots with guacamole or hummus, apples or celery with a dollop of organic peanut or almond butter, pieces of zucchini or broccoli with extra-virgin olive oil and a sprinkle of sea salt. For a light summer meal, simply serve up a plate of fresh cut vegetables and sauces.

Roast them. I love roasted vegetables. They are "fast food" for the kitchen—easy and quick. In spite of this, or maybe because of it, they always seem special. In any season, you can gather the vegetables that are in your kitchen, cut them all in bite sized pieces, season with herbs, sea salt, and oil, and pop in a hot oven. As they cook, the smell tantalizes. A few minutes later you have a feast. Roast vegetables until they are browned on the edges and soft in the center. In autumn and winter, roast cranberries and slices of winter squash, or a mixture of potatoes - sweets and russets. Look for Recipes at the end of the book.

Grill them. Our grill is used throughout the summer for easy meals and impromptu feasts. Grill asparagus, long quarters of zucchini, or fat slices of eggplant slathered with olive oil, herbs and sea salt. Skewer sweet onions, tomatoes and bell peppers to grill, then top them with a vinaigrette dressing.

Steam them. To steam a vegetable, you can use a metal or bamboo steamer, or you can just cook it in a little water. Steaming vegetables just until they are done preserves the color and many of the nutrients. A good rule of thumb for green leafy vegetables is to steam them until they are bright green. For kale and broccoli, this takes just about 5 minutes. Steam new potatoes until they are soft and add dill. Steam green beans with rosemary until they have just lost their brightness and become soft. To steam, place vegetables in a heavy pot with a tight lid. Add 1/2 - 1 inch of water. Add an herb and a little butter, ghee, or olive oil. Cover and cook it on medium heat. When steam escapes, turn the heat down to the lowest setting for a few minutes and then toss with a sprinkle of sea salt. Different vegetables may require different amounts of cooking time.

Stir-fry them. We often think of Asian foods when we think of stir-frying, but many vegetables lend themselves to this method of cooking. Stir-frying is fast and preserves many nutrients that might be lost in a slower way of cooking. Try stir-frying zucchini with dill, or red, yellow and green bell peppers with chopped jicama, sweet onion and thyme. To stir-fry, heat a stable oil like coconut or avocado oil in a large skillet or wok over high heat. You know the oil is hot enough when an added drop of water rolls and skitters across the surface. Add vegetables in small increments to preserve the heated skillet, stir and turn until vegetables are crisp-tender. Serve with a splash of soy sauce or a drizzle of olive oil and some sea salt.

SEASON WELL

When cooking vegetables, there is always a balance between showcasing the flavor of the vegetable and seasoning enough to keep the taste full and interesting. The flavor of most vegetables will benefit from the addition of one of these herbs: thyme, dill, rosemary, sage, oregano and basil. Add a little butter, ghee or olive oil to mellow and enhance the flavor of the vegetable. Add a pinch of sea salt. Do not be afraid to experiment until you find your favorite taste combinations.

MICROWAVING YOUR FOOD

Although not all the research agrees, there is mounting evidence that microwave ovens destroy vital nutrients in food whereas slower, more conventional cooking preserves the nutrients. Microwaving in plastic adds insult to injury because there is the very real possibility of chemicals from the plastic migrating into the food. While it is best not to microwave foods at all, if you are going to use the microwave, make sure to use only glass containers. Many times, preparing foods on the stove or in the oven adds only a couple of minutes to preparation time. But the resulting product is better because it is evenly heated and retains the flavors and nutrients.

ORGANIC VS. CONVENTIONAL

A few decades ago there was no need to label foods "organic." This is because most foods were organic back then. When pesticides, herbicides and chemical fertilizers were introduced, it was in the interest of increasing food production and reducing world-hunger—noble ideals to be sure. But many of these chemicals have been unleashed on our food supply without adequate testing and assurance of safety. "With more than 10,000 additives allowed in food, Pew's research found that the FDA regulatory system is plagued with systemic problems, which prevent the agency from ensuring that their use is safe.[5]"

I am often asked if I think everyone should eat organic foods exclusively. My answer is yes because our bodies were not meant to ingest pesticides, herbicides and chemical fertilizers no matter how small the amount; our bodies have enough pollutants to deal with without adding insult to injury by adding these chemicals to our diets. The long-term effects of ingesting preservatives and herbicides has not been thoroughly tested. In addition, many times otherwise "safe" chemicals can combine in the body to produce compounds that have never been tested for safety, or have been proven to be harmful.[6] So, in a perfect world, I would never touch a food that was not organically grown.

We do not live in a perfect world. Sometimes the only vegetables that are available are non-organically grown vegetables, that is, those raised without the benefit of organic practices, or those that are not certified organic. Sometimes the organic vegetables have to be transported over great distances, leaving a large environmental footprint and losing nutrients in the long journey from farm to table. Sometimes organic vegetables are prohibitively expensive. Be aware of the following when choosing between organic and conventional foods:

USDA Certified Organic: Foods that are certified organic in the United States can bear the label "USDA Certified." There are certain rules that govern foods and the land they are grown on that are labeled with this certification. First and foremost, these foods have gone through testing to verify that irradiation, sewage sludge, synthetic fertilizers, prohibited pesticides, and genetically modified organisms were not used.[7]

"Organically raised" foods are often raised by small farmers using organic practices who are not able to afford the expensive USDA certification. This is a time when it is beneficial to be involved in your community and to know your local farmers. Most farmers I know who are raising foods organically are conscientious, and will tell you honestly what practices they use in growing their fruits and vegetables. I buy these foods whenever possible to support local small farmers.

The Dirty Dozen and Clean Fifteen: Some fruits and vegetables are loaded with chemicals; others are naturally pest-resistant and do not require added chemicals. When strawberries grown with conventional farming practices are brought to market, they often contain large quantities of pesticides. This is because they are highly absorbent like sponges, and because they are too fragile to be washed thoroughly. Many crops, including apples, contain large amounts of pesticides because the pesticide is inside the fruit or vegetable and cannot be washed off. On the other hand, bugs do not generally bother onions and garlic. Even conventionally raised onions and garlic generally do not have many pesticides. The Environmental Working Group is a watchdog for the food and cosmetic industries. For a list of the most and least contaminated fruits and vegetables, go to their website. There you will find a list of fifty fruits and vegetables rated from best to worst, including the Dirty Dozen and the Clean Fifteen.[8] The Environmental Working Group updates its list yearly. They even have an app available for smart phones so you can take the list to the grocery store with you.

IRRADIATION

The Environmental Protection Agency tells us that food is irradiated to protect against harmful bacteria and food-borne pathogens. Foods are irradiated using gamma rays, electron beams or x-rays. The EPA assures us that years of experience in food irradiation has not demonstrated any identifiable health problems.[9] However, Organic Consumers Association tells a different story. They say that irradiation damages valuable nutrients in the food, and has not been thoroughly tested to determine the long term effects. They point out that irradiated foods are insufficiently marked for consumers to make an informed decision, and that irradiation discourages responsible practices amongst growers.[10]

How do you avoid irradiation? The EPA requires that irradiated food bear a label.[11] However, only the first recipient of the food sees the label. For instance, if a spice is irradiated, and then used in the manufacture of a processed food, then the processed food does not have to bear the label stating the irradiation of it's contents. At this time, the only way to insure that your foods is not irradiated is to buy USDA Certified Organic.

GMOs

Many people have heard about genetically modified organisms (GMOs), but not so many actually understand what this is. The World Health Organization defines genetically modified organisms (GMOs) as "plants or animals whose DNA has been modified in a way that could not have occurred naturally through mating or natural recombination."[12] An example of a genetically modified food is Bt corn, developed by Monsanto Corporation, which kills corn borers (a worm) by punching holes in their stomach lining. This is accomplished by splicing the DNA of the bacterium bacillus thuringiensis to corn. Every cell in the corn contains this genetic material; it cannot be washed off. While official channels maintain that this bacteria is harmless to humans, there is considerable speculation among some scientists that the genetically engineered Bt is anything but benign.[13] The biggest problem with GMOs is that their claims of safety are unproven over a significant period of time. So the human population is unwittingly participating in a huge science experiment. It is best to err on the side of caution.

There is no rule that companies have to label products containing genetically engineered foods. Many companies that are involved in the production of these foods are actively lobbying for there to be no labeling requirement and, in fact, to make it unlawful to provide any labeling regarding GMOs.

There are two ways to make sure your food contains no GMOs. The first is to buy USDA Certified Organic foods. These foods are not allowed to contain GMOs. The second is to look on the food package for the seal of the Non-GMO Certified Project™. This organization describes themselves this way: "The Non-GMO Project is a non-profit organization committed to preserving and building sources of non-GMO products, educating consumers, and providing verified non-GMO choices."[14].

CHECKLIST FOR GETTING YOUR FRUITS AND VEGETABLES

- ✓ Eat a cornucopia of healthy colors.

- ✓ Choose seasonal, locally grown produce.

- ✓ Fill half your plate with fruits and non-starchy vegetables.

- ✓ Cook and season your vegetables well to heighten your enjoyment.

- ✓ Choose USDA certified organic, or choose foods that you know were organically raised by your local farmer.

- ✓ Visit the Environmental Working Group website to see which fruits and vegetables are the most and least contaminated with regard to pesticides.

- ✓ Be aware of fruits and vegetables that are genetically modified, and steer clear of them.

step 5: stock the larder

"You are what you eat eats."
Michael Pollan[1]

MEATS AND OTHER CONTROVERSIES

Ask anyone today about their diet and they will quickly announce themselves as vegetarians (people who eschew meat), vegans (vegetarians who eat no animal products, including honey and eggs), ovo-vegetarians (vegetarians that eat eggs), lacto-vegetarians (vegetarians that eat milk products), ovo-lacto-vegetarians, pescatarians (people who call themselves vegetarian but eat fish), pollo-vegetarians (people who call themselves vegetarian but eat chicken), omnivores (people who eat plants and animals) and paleo-enthusiasts (people who try to eat a diet similar to early humans). There are people who eschew red meat, and others who will not touch a chicken but will dive into a steak. Popular reasons for diet choices in relation to meat center on health, ethics, and spirituality. Entire organizations align themselves on the basis of their members' relationship to meat. Each camp has clear reasons for their choices and research to back them up. Who, then, are we to believe?

Your health is both an important consideration and a significant indicator of which diet is best for you. Dr. Joseph Mercola believes that people fall into three nutritional types: protein, carb and mixed. Protein-types feel better when they eat significant amounts of the right type of protein, usually high-quality meats. Carb-types make the healthiest vegetarians because they have low protein requirements and feel optimally healthy when consuming mostly plant foods. Mixed-type people require a mix of high-quality protein from animal sources along with significant portions of plant foods.[2] My own experience with clients confirms this. I find that, while some people thrive on a vegetarian diet, others suffer ill effects from going long periods of time without high-quality meats in their diet.

I always ask if someone has chosen vegetarianism because of health-related, ethical or spiritual reasons. If the reason is their health, I explain to them why the saturated fats found in grass-fed and pastured meats are extremely healthy, and I encourage them to try these meats to see if their health improves. If the reason is ethics, I encourage them to research how the ethics of raising animals in a factory feedlot differs from raising animals that have true access to fresh grass and sunshine throughout their lives. It is possible to eat meat and still support the humane and responsible treatment of animals.

COWS 'N PIGS

The first time I met my local meat farmer, Tracy, I underestimated him. I had wandered into a market and found a counter with a sign advertising "Grass-Fed Beef." There was Tracy in his signature overalls. I had encountered a number of people who thought they knew what grass-fed beef was, but were misinformed. I began quizzing him.

"Tell me about your grass-fed beef. Do your cows have access to pasture?"

"Yes ma'am."

"Do you ever feed them corn?"

"No ma'am."

"What do you feed them the last three months before slaughter?"

"They eat grass."

By now Tracy was grinning. He could see where this conversation was going.

"So they are fed grass their entire lives?"

"Yes ma'am."

"And you never feed them grain?"

"No ma'am."

It turns out that Tracy studied under Joe Salatin, who some call the father of grass-fed beef in America. Tracy knows how to properly produce delicious, healthy, grass-fed beef and pastured pork and chicken. He treats his animals humanely. While this is important from an ethical viewpoint, it is also necessary for the meat to be the healthiest. Fear experienced by an animal during its slaughter significantly elevates the level of stress hormones in its meat—adrenaline, cortisol, and other steroids. Scientists believe that consumption of these hormones is worrisome.[3]

There is a tremendous difference in the quality of beef between humanely-raised, grass-fed cows from a small farm and cows which are raised in CAFOs (Concentrated Animal Feedlot Operations). These CAFOs are "large-scale mechanized mega-farms where hundreds of thousands of cows, pigs, chickens and turkeys are fed and fattened for market, all within the confines of enclosed buildings or crowded outdoor lots."[4] Cows raised in these factory farms are given little room to move throughout their lifetimes. They are kept in cages the size of their bodies and they stand in their own excrement. Most are unable to lie down. Since these animals are highly stressed, their meat contains large amounts of stress hormones. "And, like many big industries, factory farms are major contributors to air, water and land pollution."[5]

Beef from these cows contributes to inflammation in humans because of its high amount of omega-6 fatty acid. This is the result of feeding the cows corn over their lifetimes. Since corn is not the natural food for a cow, the animals have to be fed antibiotics to keep them healthy enough to survive until slaughter. Some 80% of all antibiotics sold in the United States are used for livestock and poultry. Daily use of antibiotics in animal feed causes antibiotic-resistant bacteria to thrive, and this creates a public health hazard.[6]

Contrast this with cattle that are raised on a small farm, and are allowed to forage for grasses, the natural food for cattle. Not only do they have a better life, but the resulting meat is healthier. Beef that is grass-fed has up to four times the amount of inflammation-busting omega-3 fat than is found in grain-fed beef. And, since the cattle live better lives, their beef contains less stress hormones. Cattle that eat grass their entire lives are leaner. The best part? Properly prepared grass-fed beef tastes cleaner and better.

It is important to know that organic is not the same as grass-fed. "These products come from animals who were fed organically grown grain, but who typically still spent most of their lives (or in the case of dairy cows perhaps their whole lives) in feedlots."[5] This means that the meat from these organically raised cows can still contain inflammatory fats and stress hormones.

Like cows, pigs can be raised in a CAFO, or on a small family farm. And like cows, their living conditions and food supply determine the quality of the pork that arrives on your dinner table. Animals that are raised on a farm and given good food and access to pasture produce meat and fat that is far healthier than industrially-farmed animals. Pigs are naturally omnivorous foragers, happily eating a variety of fresh vegetables, fruits and meat. If they are fed a diet similar to the foods they would forage for, their meat will contain a full complement of healthy vitamins and minerals. However, factory-farmed animals are generally fed powdered feed so that they will fatten quickly. The resulting meat is lower in nutritional value and is laced with antibiotics.[7]

THE SKINNY ON HEALTHY FATS

In Chapter 3 I mentioned some good oils—coconut, olive and avocado. This is only the list of healthy vegetable fats. Does the phrase "healthy fats" sound like an oxymoron? For years fats have been vilified, especially saturated fats. Surprisingly, some saturated fats are healthy, and even necessary.

Our bodies need fat. Fat helps to regulate a whole host of bodily processes. Fats provide energy, regulate hormones, carry vitamins to cells, increase mineral absorption, and are building blocks for cell membranes—just to name a few of the benefits. Your brain, in particular, needs saturated fats to function properly. Eating some healthy fat is necessary to keep from getting hungry.

The point at which fats start breaking down in cooking is called the "smoke point." When a fat is heated past its smoke point, the fat begins to break down, releasing free radicals and a substance called acrolein, the chemical that gives burnt foods their acrid flavor and aroma.[8] The best fats for cooking are fats that have a high smoke point. These include coconut oil, avocado oil, butter and ghee, and saturated animal fats.

Butter and Ghee—Once thought to be unhealthy, butter contains nutrients that are hard to find elsewhere, and it is now being considered a superfood. Butter contains healthy vitamins and minerals as well as a perfect balance of omega-3 and omega-6 fatty acids. It also contains butyric acid which is important in colon health. The best butter comes from grass-fed cows and is raw. If you cannot find this, look for organic butter, or organic cultured butter.

Ghee is traditionally used in Indian cooking, and is better for frying because it has a higher smoke point than butter. It can be made easily by bringing butter to a boil and skimming away the milk solids. (See the Recipes chapter.) Ghee can be stored at room temperature. Because it contains no lactose or casein, it can be tolerated by people with dairy allergies.

Margarine really has nothing in common with butter, except that it looks similar—thanks to yellow food coloring—and is found in the same refrigerated case as butter. Margarine is produced from oils through a process called hydrogenation. In this process, oils are extracted from seeds using high temperature, pressure and the chemical hexane. The raw oils are then mixed with toxic nickel or other metals that serve as a catalyst for the hydrogenation process. The oils are put under high pressure to facilitate the hydrogenation process. Hydrogenation causes the formation of trans fats. The remaining mass is steamed again and bleached to get rid of the grey color. Synthetic vitamins and flavors are mixed in. Oddly enough, the food coloring is natural because artificial colors are not allowed in this thoroughly artificial product.[9] Margarine has no place in a healthy diet.

Saturated animal fats—Lard, beef fat and other animal fats have gotten a bad rap. Doctors and advertisements warn us away from fats from pork and beef. So it may come as a surprise to learn that saturated animal fats can be healthy. Mary G. Enig PhD, co-founder of the Weston A. Price Foundation, offers the following evidence: Heart disease was rare in America before 1920. However, during the next 40 years, the incidence of heard disease rose dramatically. By the 1950s heart disease was the leading cause of death among Americans. As of the year 2000, heart disease caused 40 percent of all deaths. Yet during that period (1910 - 1970), the proportion of animal fat in the American diet declined and cholesterol increased only 1 percent. What changed? During this same period, the percentage of dietary vegetable oils in the form of margarine, shortening and refined oils increased about 400 percent and the consumption of sugar and processed foods increased about 60 percent.[10]

As with most foods, the source matters. Fat from factory-farmed animals is loaded with toxins and inflammation-causing fatty acids. But fat from grass-fed cows and lard from pastured pork contain a host of health promoting ingredients.

Lard contains 48% mono saturated fat, 40% saturated fat, and 12% polyunsaturated fats. The fats in pastured lard are, believe it or not, heart healthy. Lard has a high smoke point and so is good for frying. Lard found at a regular grocery store is likely from factory-farmed animals unless it states otherwise. I only purchase lard from my farmer who also raises pastured pigs. Tracy usually has the lard already rendered and ready to use. Lard contains cholesterol which, contrary to popular opinion, is a necessary component of your diet and does not set you up for heart disease.[11]

A GOOD EGG

As with other farm products, there is a vast difference between the quality of pasture-farmed chicken meat and eggs and those produced on factory farms. Pastured chickens are humanely raised, out of doors, with access to pasture and sunshine, and in an area where they can forage for their natural diet. In addition, they are fed wholesome grains. Chickens require an additional grain supplement to give them the nutrients necessary to be healthy. The bugs and worms in their diet mean that the resulting meat and eggs will naturally be higher in good omega-3 fatty acids. The egg yolks will be darker and richer, and will taste better. Pastured egg shells may come in shades of brown, white and aqua. The color is an indication of the breed of chicken and has no bearing on quality. The best source for finding high-quality poultry and eggs is a local farmer who raises pastured chickens. You can also find them in natural grocery stores. Expect to pay more. But for what you pay, you are ensured that the chicken was humanely raised, and that you are getting the best nutritional benefit from your purchase. Find local farmers by visiting your farmers' market.

Eggs are confusing these days. Prices range from quite cheap to incredibly high, and the labels make it difficult to understand what you are really paying for. Here are some of the differences:

Plain eggs—usually the least expensive. These eggs are from regular chickens who live their lives in extremely crowded and unsanitary conditions in cages that are stacked on top of each other in factory warehouse farms. Because they are so stressed from their environment, the chickens tend to peck at each other. To prevent damage from pecking, often their beaks and wings are painfully clipped. They are fed cheap feed that is nutritionally deficient. The eggs
they produce are a far cry, nutritionally, from what eggs are supposed to be.

Cage-free—You might visualize chickens roaming around in free conditions when you see "cage-free", but this simply means that the chickens are not kept in cages. They still are likely to live in crowded, stressful conditions and have their beaks and wings clipped.

Free Range—Again, you might picture chickens with freedom here, but "free range" simply means that there is a small door somewhere in the warehouse to let the chickens have access to the out of doors. "Out of doors" might be a three-foot square dirt patch for an entire warehouse of chickens. Like "cage free," "free range" can be deceiving.

USDA Certified Organic—Chickens are fed certified organic feed and are likely to have had exposure to some sunlight. This is an improvement because at least you are not getting pesticides and GMOs in your food. The Certified Organic label does not address the conditions that the chickens live in or whether or not they are treated humanely.

Vegetarian feed—This may sound like a wonderful thing, but chickens are supposed to eat bugs and worms. An entirely vegetarian diet means corn and soy. This is not the healthiest diet for a chicken and therefore does not produce the healthiest eggs.

Omega-3 enriched—again, this may sound great, but eggs naturally contain omega-3 when the chickens are able to eat bugs and worms. The flax seed usually used in the feed when eggs are omega-3 enriched is not a natural part of the chicken's diet.

Pasture-raised eggs—these are the eggs you want to purchase for the greatest health benefit.

A CASE FOR DAIRY

A generation ago, milk was consumed with little thought of whether or not it was healthy. Of course it was healthy—the American Dairy Association, along with milk-mustachioed celebrities, told us so. Since then, milk has become another vilified and confusing food. We worry about the cholesterol, and the possibility of added hormones and antibiotics. And, are we as humans supposed to drink milk from animals at all? Healthy milk is available, but what constitutes "healthy" may surprise you.

For years, millions of people, concerned about saturated fats and cholesterol, have eschewed whole milk. As I mentioned earlier, saturated fat is not the problem we thought it was. Whole milk is simply milk that still has the butter, or fat, in it. Drinking the whole milk gives you a balance of needed fat-soluble nutrients A, D, E and K, and the right amount of protein. Skim milk, on the other hand, is a manufactured product. Because there is no fat in skim milk, something has to be done to disguise the unappealing bluish, translucent color, thin texture and the lack of flavor. So, milk solids are added back to skim milk to give it color and flavor. These highly processed milk solids contain oxidized cholesterol which contributes to inflammation in the body.[12] The resulting product is low on nutritional value, since most of the vital nutrients in milk are in the fat. And it contains a double dose of the potentially allergen-causing protein, casein.

Milk only contains a full measure of vitamins A, E and K when cows graze on grass in pastures, and D is produced when cows have access to sunshine. Milk from the grocery store used to have synthetic vitamin D2 added; these days some manufacturers have switched to vitamin D3. The resulting product is labeled "vitamin D enriched." Humans need vitamin D3. D2 provides only a very limited benefit and can be toxic in high doses.[13]

The healthiest milk comes, unaltered, from a healthy pasture-raised cow. Raw milk is controversial from the government's point of view, and the sale of it is illegal in some states. But no one can deny that raw milk has sustained humanity for generations untold, and continues to be a safe, life-giving whole food in many less-developed areas of the world. The healthiest grocery store option is whole milk from a small dairy where the cows have had ample access to pastures. If these small family farms can assure you that their milk is organic, that is all the better.

HOW SAFE IS FISH?

Fish is an excellent source of lean protein, and some fish, especially salmon, is an excellent place to get your health-promoting omega-3 fats. But a lot of people, myself included, have tended to avoid fish because of the scare about mercury and toxins. How do you know that the fish you are eating is really safe? There are some guidelines for choosing fish that is safe.

Wild-caught vs farmed: In general, wild-caught fish are safer than farmed. Farmed fish fall prey to some of the same problems of overcrowding and toxic feed that plague other factory-farmed animals. Salmon that are farmed contain pesticides (for sea lice), synthetic pigments (because the flesh would be an unappetizing grey without it), a higher fat content and a lower ratio of omega-3 fatty acids. They are fed antibiotics because they cannot survive the crowded pen conditions without them. In addition, waste from these marine farms pollutes the water.[14]

Even wild-caught salmon may be suspect because many of the lower-priced, wild-caught fish are actually hatched and farmed for half their life and then set free before they are captured again as adults in the wild. True wild-caught salmon comes at a premium price. Your best bet? Save up to be able to afford truly wild-caught salmon.[15]

Brierley Wright, M.S., R.D. suggests eating the following healthy fish:

- Albacore tuna that has been poll-caught or troll-caught. Smaller fish are caught in this way, so there is less mercury build up.
- Wild-caught salmon and sardines.

- Farmed oysters and rainbow trout, which can be farmed without hurting the environment.

- Freshwater Coho salmon, which are farmed in tanks. This is the first and only kind of farmed salmon to get a "Super Green" rating.

She also suggests avoiding these fishes:

- Bluefin tuna and Chilean Sea Bass (threatened species).

- Grouper (high mercury content and prone to over-fishing).

- Monkfish and Orange Roughy (prone to over-fishing).

- Farmed salmon (for reasons above).[16]

And what about tilapia? Dr Andrew Weil reports that tilapia contain very little omega-3 fats, and a substantial amount of inflammation-producing omega-6 fats. This means that, while eating tilapia may not be dangerous, there are better choices out there.[17]

CHECKLIST: RESOURCES FOR MEATS, FISH, EGGS, AND DAIRY

- ✔ Farmer's Markets are good places to meet local beef, pork, chicken and diary farmers.

- ✔ Natural grocery stores are more likely to carry pastured meats and eggs, as well as safe fish from sustainable sources.

- ✔ Specialty markets are generally more knowledgeable and discerning about their sources than regular grocery stores.

- ✔ Buy directly from the farmer. Many small farmers will have extra meat, milk or eggs for sale. Inquire at farmers' markets and local markets to find local farmers.

- ✔ Grow your own. Raising chickens is a popular hobby.

step 6:
have your
just desserts

"The way you treat yourself sets
the standard for others."

Sonya Friedman

THE THING ABOUT SWEETS

It is universal—almost everybody loves the taste of something sweet. What is it about sugar that we love so much? Even though we know we absolutely do NOT need that piece of pie, or the big-gulp soda, or the second serving of ice cream, why do we reach for something sweet anyway? Why do we crave sweets? The answer to that lies in ancient history. Our early ancestors were more likely to survive if they valued the taste of sugar and the quick energy it provided. For those same ancestors, the fact that sugar caused weight gain would have been an additional factor favorable to their survival.

Fast forward to today, and those same survival mechanisms seem to be working against us. We have so many more sweets available to us than humans did in the early years. In those days, the supply of sweets were limited. Back then, gorging on a newly-found stash of honey or fruit meant survival. Today, downing a newly-found stash of chocolate candy does not produce the same positive payback.

AN ABBREVIATED HISTORY OF SUGAR

Around 510 B.C., when the Persian emperor Darius I invaded India, he found a reed that he thought contained honey. This sugarcane was burned in religious ceremonies, eaten, and used for medicine. Ancient Greeks and Romans brought the cane from India to grow and to use as a medicine. From there it spread throughout Europe as an expensive spice reserved for the very wealthy. The Crusaders brought knowledge of how to grow sugarcane back to Europe. Christopher Columbus brought sugarcane plants to the Caribbean.[1]

Why is the history of sugar important? To show that humans did not evolve eating pure sugar. Before sugar was invented, humans only had access to natural sugars in fruits, honey or sweet vegetables. If we follow this brief history up to today, we will find that sugar consumption (including high fructose corn syrup) has gone from zero, once upon a time, to 156 pounds per person per year.[2] Picture 31 five-pound bags of sugar lined up. That is an average of 41 teaspoons per day, or well over a half a cup. Now, I certainly do not eat that much sugar, and you may not either, which means that someone else is eating even more than the average. No wonder we are sick!

ALL THAT SUGAR

According to the Health.com, the following foods contribute the highest percentage of total added sugar to the diets of Americans:[3]

- Regular soft drinks: 33%

- Sugars and candy: 16%

- Cakes, cookies and pies: 13%

- Fruit drinks: 10%

- Dairy desserts and milk products: 8%

- Other grains: 6%

It is interesting that a whopping 33 percent of our sugar consumption is in sweet drinks. To get a clear picture, calculate your sugar like this: One small cube of sugar is equal to four grams. Grab a box from your shelf and look at the nutrition label on the back. Find the amount of sugar in grams on the item, and divide that number by four. The result is the number of sugar cubes in one serving of that item.

High doses of sugar can have devastating effects on our health. Here is a partial list.[4]

- Sugar causes inflammation.

- Sugar can suppress the immune system.

- Sugar can cause hyperactivity, anxiety, difficulty concentrating, and crankiness, and it can worsen symptoms of ADHD.

- Sugar interferes with the absorption of minerals.

- Sugar can cause or contribute to obesity, arthritis, asthma, heart disease, multiple sclerosis, gout, depression, Alzheimer's disease, tooth decay, Crohn's disease, ulcerative colitis, Candida albicans infections, and eczema.

- Sugar can cause cancer: gastric, pancreatic, gastrointestinal, prostate and laryngeal, to name a few.

- Sugar raises cholesterol and lowers high-density lipoproteins (the "good" cholesterol).

- Sugar can slow food's travel time through the gastrointestinal tract.

- Sugar can contribute to diabetes by causing a decrease in insulin sensitivity.

HIGH FRUCTOSE CORN SYRUP

Much of the sugar that is being consumed these days, especially in drinks, is in the form of high fructose corn syrup (HFCS.) HFCS was invented in the late 1950s and went into commercial production in the late 1960s. At the time it was considered to be similar to sugar. We now know that it is not. HFCS has a higher percentage of fructose than sugar does, and our body processes it differently. "Unlike excess glucose, which passes through our digestive tract and is excreted, 100 percent of fructose that is consumed is taken up by the liver. Once there, fructose causes increased fat deposition in the abdominal cavity and increased blood levels of triglycerides—both of which are risk factors for heart disease and diabetes."[5]

Dr. Mark Hyman contends that there are two real issues:

- "We are consuming HFCS and sugar in pharmacologic quantities never before experienced in human history–140 pounds a year versus 20 teaspoons a year 10,000 years ago.

- "High fructose corn syrup is always found in very poor-quality foods that are nutritionally vacuous and filled with all sorts of other disease promoting compounds, fats, salt, chemicals, and even mercury."[6]

The bottom line is this: Deciding to quit eating and drinking high fructose corn syrup could have a profound positive impact on your health. Continuing will have a decidedly negative impact.

ARTIFICIAL SWEETENERS

The word is out—eat less sugar. In response, people have flocked to artificial sweeteners such as aspartame (diet colas and Equal®), saccharin (Sweet 'n Low®), and sucralose (Splenda®). Officially, according to the National Cancer Institute, there is no clear evidence that artificial sweeteners on the market in the U.S. are related to cancer risk in humans.[7] However, one long-term study correlates drinking one or more cans of diet soda with an increased risk of cancer.[8] Another study links consumption of artificial sweeteners to glucose intolerance.[9] Yet another connects artificial sweeteners to impaired cognitive memory function.[10] While all of this sounds rather technical, it is making a clear point: artificial sweeteners are not health-promoting. Artificial sweeteners are not real food.

NATURAL SWEETENERS

The good news is that you can have some sweet foods in your life. There are sweeteners that, when eaten in small portions, can be part of a healthy diet. These include honey, maple syrup and molasses. Because they are natural and not processed chemicals, your body knows what to do with them. The queen bee in this list is raw honey. Raw honey has never been heated, or pasteurized, so it still contains natural enzymes. It is antiviral and antibacterial and has been used for many health maladies including allergies, diarrhea, wound healing and acid reflux.[11] Raw honey that is local to your area may also help with seasonal allergies. Look for raw honey at a natural grocery store. Maple syrup and molasses are unprocessed natural sweeteners that contain some minerals and antioxidants. Look for 100% raw honey, maple syrup, and molasses, and be sure you aren't getting products that are cut with high fructose corn syrup. Remember to enjoy in small quantities because too many concentrated sweeteners in any form can be detrimental to your health.

Stevia comes in many forms, from natural ground leaves, to highly processed sweeteners that contain stevia mixed with other substances that may not be good for you at all. For instance, Truvia® contains processed stevia mixed with erythritol, among other ingredients. Erythritol is a sugar alcohol that can cause digestive distress and diarrhea. Stevia is often highly processed to remove the bitter component. It is important to read the label since most sweeteners labeled "stevia" have other ingredients. So some brands of this "natural" sweetener may not be natural at all. It is possible to purchase whole, unprocessed stevia leaves but oddly, the FDA has not approved this form as a sweetener, only the more processed versions.

Fruit is nature's dessert. When we eat fruit, we are also getting a host of nutrients and healthy fiber in addition to the sugar. The fiber slows the absorption of the natural fruit sugar, so there is less likely to be a spike in insulin as a result. Fruit juice has had most, or all, of the fiber removed, and can cause a spike in insulin. Your best bet is to enjoy a couple of servings a day of whole fruit, rather than drinking fruit juice.

HOW TO TAME YOUR CRAVINGS

Our bodies are simply not made for the concentrated simple sugars we often encounter in processed products. Overconsumption of simple carbohydrates triggers insulin production which, in turn, triggers hypoglycemia. When this happens, our blood sugar becomes low and we crave sweets because our body needs a spike in glucose. It is a vicious cycle.

Long before we had access to concentrated sugars, people associated a sweet taste with safe, non-poisonous foods. They satisfied cravings and with foods like fruit, squash, tubers, roots and grains. This is still the best way to satisfy your cravings today—indulge in sweet vegetables like sweet potatoes and winter squash, as well as fruits. Then your body will not cry out for the concentrated sweetness you find in processed sweets. If you have been used to eating a lot of sugar, it will take awhile to wean yourself from sweets.

Make sure you include sweet vegetables and fruits in your food daily, especially while you are breaking sugar's hold on you.

Sometimes your cravings for sweets have nothing to do with food. You may be thirsty. Drink a glass of water. Sometimes a craving is your body asking you to take a walk. You may need some sleep. Sleep deprived people eat more. You may be bored. Take a break and do something interesting and fun for a few minutes and see if your craving is still with you. Your taste buds may simply be craving a new flavor that could be satisfied with some new and interesting food. Or you may be distressed. It is better to find the source of the unhappiness and correct that.

FYI

The phrase "just desserts" does not really exist. The actual phrase, "just deserts," means that someone gets what they deserve, good or bad. So, deserve your dessert. If you give up mindlessly eating sugar and sweets and become savvy about the sweets you eat, you get a reward: the ability to have dessert without guilt on occasion. Activist author Michael Pollen has some sage advise about eating sweets. "Eat all the junk food you want as long as you cook it yourself."[12] Think about it. If you had to prepare all of the sweets you eat from scratch, would you really have to worry about overeating sweets? Just do not let yourself eat the whole pan of homemade brownies in one sitting! The quote at the beginning of this chapter bears a moment of thought as well. Are you treating yourself well when you mindlessly ingest too much sugar? Treat yourself like you matter by protecting your health.

10 SWEET SNACKS TO SATISFY YOUR SWEET TOOTH

- ✅ apple with almond butter

- ✅ frozen grapes

- ✅ bars (Lara Bars, Kits Organic Bars, protein bars.) Choose a brand that has an ingredients list you can understand.

- ✅ apple, peach, or banana chips

- ✅ sugar snap peas

- ✅ rice cakes with raw honey

- ✅ yogurt with raw honey & nuts

- ✅ a piece of dark chocolate

- ✅ frozen mangos, right out of the bag

- ✅ peaches with cottage cheese

step 7: prepare simple fare

"Cooking is like love. It should be entered into with abandon, or not at all."

Julia Child

LOVE TO COOK

There was a time when everyone knew how to cook. It is what you did if you wanted to eat. These days the science of nutrition has become quite technical. We are finding out a lot of new information about how food affects health. But there is so much information and misinformation out there that people feel overwhelmed. Suddenly we do not feel competent to put a meal on the table. What if I get it wrong? What if I get the carb ratio out of whack, or serve too much protein, or not enough, or the wrong kind? We have lost confidence in our own ability to nourish and sustain ourselves.

We rush. And in all of that rushing around, we move the nourishing and caring for our bodies to the bottom of the to-do list. Cooking well and eating well is seen as a weekend treat rather than a necessity. We have abdicated our health to pre-cooked and processed foods from corporations whose bottom line is profit, not healthy food. One of the most profound ways to become proactive in your own health is to take up the life-sustaining craft of cooking. This participation in your own health is available to anyone with a pot and a bit of food. Preparing a meal can nourish the soul the way food nourishes the body.

This is the step where we put all the information into perspective. So that you are not completely overwhelmed, begin simply. I have helped with this by providing a few simple recipes in the last chapter of the book. Each of the recipes has only a few ingredients and can be the basis for a satisfying meal.

Expect to make mistakes. Not everything you cook will turn out flawlessly, at least not the first time. When I make a new recipe, it is rarely perfect. I may make it several times, adjusting and writing notes in the margins of my cookbook each time before I am satisfied. Sometimes a recipe does not suit me at all and, after making it once, I never make it again. There was the time when I attempted to make turkey chili. It tasted distinctly of bird, and not in a good way. My daughter remembers the Thanksgiving gravy that resembled phlegm. There was the pot of green beans I put on the stove and then forgot. I was about twenty minutes from home in my car when I remembered it. (Do not try this one!) There was the stuff that was supposed to gel but never did, and the other stuff that seized up like rubber. I could go on . . .

The best cooks can cook without a recipe, instinctively knowing how to adjust proportions of ingredients and add a pinch of this or that until the outcome is stupendous. Paradoxically, the way to learn how to do this is to cook with recipes as you learn what works and what does not. As you make a recipe more than once, begin to adjust the seasoning just to see what a dash of Tabasco sauce adds, or a pinch of thyme, or an extra clove of garlic. Over time, cooking can become instinctive and simple, and the process can be tremendously satisfying. If I am honest, I will admit that somedays I do not feel much satisfaction in cooking. On those days it is a chore. But even then I am grateful to have the competence to put a quick and nourishing meal on the table.

So think of this as play. Put on some good music; don a fancy apron, or a funky one, or a practical one. Recruit a helper and have a great conversation while you cook. Pour a glass of wine if that will spark your creativity, and celebrate the time you spend in the kitchen.

INSPIRATION

I love cookbooks. My favorite cookbooks not only contain delicious whole food recipes, but beautiful pictures. My favorite recipes are the ones that are simple to make, delicious, and beautiful on the plate. Often a new cookbook is the basis for experimentation for an entire season. I will bring a cookbook home and try a bunch of the recipes before I move on to another book. Invariably, a few of those recipes will become new favorites. And when I need new inspiration, or want to learn to cook in a new way, I am off to the bookstore or the internet again, dreaming of the next new cookbook. Here is a short list of my current favorites:

At Home In the Whole Foods Kitchen[1]—This cookbook is a new favorite. Amy Chaplin is a whole foods chef who creates inspiring, healthy dishes in her beautiful, airy kitchen. I love the variety of delicious healthy vegetarian foods found in this cookbook even though I am not vegetarian. The pictures are gorgeous. Try: Cherry Coconut Granola.

Everyday Food: Great Food Fast[2]—This collection of recipes from Martha Stewart Living Magazine has been my go to for fast easy cooking for years. Most meals are simple to cook and worthy of serving to company. Try: Thai-Style Steak Salad in the summer.

Paleo Comfort Food[3]—My cooking is influenced by the Paleo movement, but I do not subscribe to this philosophy 100%. That said, these recipes by Julie and Charles Mayfield have been the inspiration for many delicious meals. Try: Bangers and Mash.

Mark Bittman's Kitchen Express[4]—I love this short and sweet cookbook of inspired dishes. None have a formal recipe. Mark shows you how to toss a few real food ingredients together to create something quick and memorable. Try: Broiled Brussels Sprouts with Hazelnuts.

The web also has thousands upon thousands of recipes. Need a Middle-Eastern lentil recipe? Google "Middle-Eastern lentil recipes." Among the hundreds that you will find, decide which one seems to suit you best. Need a recipe that calls for the chicken legs you got on sale? My Google search for "recipe chicken legs" turned up the following: Caramelized Baked Chicken Legs, Spicy Roasted Chicken Legs, Braised Chicken Legs and Roasted Chicken Legs with Potatoes and Kale, just to name a few. Maybe you have never heard of a cooking ingredient, such as star anise. Or maybe you are out of baking powder and need a substitution. A web search will give you answers in a couple of seconds. As you become more familiar with real foods, you will gravitate toward healthier whole food recipes. Soon you will find yourself at ease in your real-foods kitchen.

A GOOD POT

May I ask you a personal question? How is your cookware? Are you still using cast-offs from your dorm days? Your cookware really is important, and can make all the difference in creating safe, delicious food that nourishes. Good cookware is an investment in your health. Cookware can be made from a variety of materials, only some of which are healthy. Other materials can damage your health. The best materials conduct heat well and do not react with your food. The worst cookware will burn food easily or transfer toxins into the food you eat. Choose stainless steel, true ceramic or enameled cast iron for non-reactive cookware. Stay away from aluminum cookware since it transfers aluminum to your food. Aluminum is sometimes implicated in Alzheimer's and other neurological diseases.

Also avoid non-stick cookware. Teflon®, when heated to high temperatures, emits toxic fumes. Sometimes aluminum cookware is coated with a polymer that contains ceramic powder. This is also called "ceramic," but is not true ceramic all the way through the pot. Because of the polymer, which can wear off over time, this is not the best choice. It is, however, better than uncoated aluminum. Discard any cookware that is pitted or, if coated, peeling.

I have a variety of cookware, but there are four pots and pans that get used daily in my house. These are a good starting point for your real-foods kitchen:

Skillet—Begin your cookware collection with a skillet that conducts heat well. Cast iron and carbon steel are the best conductors of heat for frying. Iron and carbon steel need to be seasoned before the first use. Do this according to the manufacturer's directions. To keep the layers of seasoning intact, wash in hot water with no soap and dry after use, then wipe a small amount of oil over the surface. It is best not to use iron and carbon steel for cooking acidic foods like tomatoes since the metal in the skillet can react with acids. Enameled cast iron solves this problem. If you use enameled cast iron, choose a good brand like Le Creuset® so that the enameled coating will last longer.

2 or 3 Quart Saucepan—This is the pan I choose for steaming vegetables and cooking sauces. Choose a pan with a tight-fitting lid in a non-reactive material like ceramic or stainless steel. The best stainless steel pans come with an aluminum plate on the bottom to conduct heat evenly. You will be more likely to burn your food in a stainless steel pan without the aluminum plate. You can also choose an enamel-coated iron pan. If you only have one saucepan, make it a 3-quart pan since many recipes will require this size. I have both 2 and 3-quart saucepans and use them often.

6 to 10 Quart Stockpot—I use my stockpot often to cook a big batch of soup or chili to freeze. Your stockpot should be made of the same kinds of non-reactive metals as your smaller saucepan.

Baking Sheet—A 13" x 17" rimmed stainless steel baking pan gets used in my kitchen almost daily.

COOKS' TOOLS

Kitchen drawers are often stuffed with gadgetry, but high-quality cook's tools are sometimes surprisingly absent. Without good cooking tools, your adventures in healthy eating will be frustrating and difficult. Buy excellent quality tools, and you will be rewarded with a cooking experience that is easier and more satisfying. Here are the top tools on my list:

Cutting Utensils—You will need three knives: a paring knife, a chef's knife, and a serrated knife. The paring knife has a short, sharp blade for peeling and cutting up fruits and vegetables. The chef's knife is a large, wide-blade knife that is used in a rocking motion for chopping. The serrated knife has a wavy edge and is good for cutting soft foods like tomatoes, bread and roast beef. Also invest in two cutting boards - a bamboo or wooden board for fruits and vegetables, and a composite board for meats. A vegetable peeler is a wonderful timesaver, and a pair of kitchen shears is indispensable for cutting meats.

Basic Cooks' Tools—If you are just beginning to cook, get yourself a set of basic kitchen cooks' tools in stainless steel. Then as you try new recipes, treat yourself to the correct tools for the recipes. My short-list of cooks' tools includes: a spatula, tongs, a stirring spoon, a slotted spoon, a long-handled cooking fork, a mesh strainer, a soup ladle, a wire whisk, a 2-cup glass measure and measuring spoons.

Appliances—My list of electric kitchen utensils is short. Even in a minimalist kitchen, I would recommend a blender or food processor. I also use a crockpot often. If you have a stock pot, you can forgo the crockpot. I love my stick blender (sometimes called an immersion blender) because it is the fastest way to blend creamy soups.

Food Storage—In general, I do not like plastic containers because they can leach chemicals into food. Xenoestrogens are endocrine disrupters which mimic estrogen in the body. They cause health problems for both men and women. Plasticizers, the chemicals that make plastic soft and pliable, contain these xenoestrogens.[5] The softer the plastic, the more plasticizers it contains. Plastic wrap on a roll is one of the worst offenders. We are exposed to these xenoestrogens everywhere in our daily lives. Bisphenol A (BPA) is one chemical of concern. It is found in epoxy resins which are used in coating the interior of food cans, and polycarbonate plastics which are used in making water bottles, among other items. Research has shown that it can seep into food from these containers. While the FDA says it is safe at very low levels, it is a concern because of possible health effects on the brain, behavior and prostate gland of fetuses, infants and children.[6]

One way you can make a difference is in your kitchen is to choose to store your food in glass containers. These can be containers collected from foods you have purchased in glass, or they can be pint or quart canning jars. Pyrex makes glass storage containers in a variety of useful shapes and sizes. These containers have plastic lids, so it is best to leave some airspace at the top of the container. If you do need to purchase plastic, look for "BPA free." This is helpful, but the containers are still composed of plasticizers. Do not heat food in the microwave in plastic or place it in plastic containers while it is still hot.

PREPARE SIMPLE FARE

You have done your homework, made a plan, gathered your food and set up your kitchen to cook uncomplicated and nourishing meals. Now it is time to begin. Here is a checklist for simple, inspired cooking.

- ✔ Learn to love to cook with a sense of adventure.

- ✔ Start with something easy.

- ✔ Be willing to be an imperfect cook. Laugh at your cooking mistakes — they make great stories.

- ✔ Be willing to experiment with new flavors.

- ✔ Look for inspiration in the form of a simple recipe.

- ✔ Gather real, whole foods, herbs, oils, and spices that nourish your body and tantalize your palate.

- ✔ Prepare your food with good cooks' tools.

- ✔ Enjoy the experience of cooking.

step 8:
eat well

"Pull up a chair. Take a taste. Come join us. Life is so endlessly delicious."

Ruth Reichl

AT TABLE

There is a scene at the beginning of the movie **Captain Ron**[1] where the wife, a busy architect, has laid a set of house plans on the kitchen table. The son comes in, pours himself a glass of milk, and then spills it all over the house plans. When the woman sees the mess, she wails, "WHO was THOUGHTLESS enough to put FOOD on the kitchen table?" And so it goes for many families. Those who still put meals on the table each day are few and far between.

This is a big deal—a really big deal! The National Center on Addiction and Substance Abuse at Columbia University (CASAColumbia) says that "Our surveys have consistently found a relationship between children having frequent dinners with their parents and a decreased risk of their smoking, drinking or using other drugs, and that parental engagement fostered around the dinner table is one of the most potent tools to help parents raise healthy, drug-free children. Simply put: frequent family dinners make a big difference."[2] At the family dinner table, children learn that they are expected to eat with some semblance of manners. They learn to participate in conversation. They learn that conversation is enjoyable, and that people have interesting stories to tell.

Relationships formed at the table are deep and lasting.

We like to think that when we go to a restaurant, there is someone in the back preparing our meal with care and appreciation. My daughter has worked in the restaurant industry. She is very familiar with the fact that meals in restaurants are prepared by harried and overworked cooks who have no interest in the food other than to preserve their jobs. She reports that she has seen a lot of screaming and mayhem going on in the back of the restaurant while you are in the dining area waiting for your meal. She speaks from experience when she says that foods in many restaurants are not prepared with love. Does it really matter that a meal is prepared with love and care? I think so. When someone you love makes you chicken soup while you are sick, it has a certain something, a quality of love that you do not get from a can or from fast-food. Ayurveda is a traditional system of healing in India that dates back thousands of years. Ayurvedic cooking subscribes to the belief that "preparing a meal with a positive intention [and] love . . . makes it even more potent and rich with healing properties."[3]

When my kids used to bring home their friends for dinner, the friends were surprised that we sat down to dinner. They were surprised because there was a meal on the table that everyone ate together, and that our kids actually had a conversation with the adults. While we ate, there were no cell phones, no iPods®, no headphones, and no TV. More than once we heard, "But we never do that at our house!" I believe that conversation at the dinner table with young children paves the way for important, and possibly difficult, conversations as they grow through the teen years and into adulthood. And, these conversation skills translate directly into the ability to converse with future teachers, marriage partners, friends, and business associates.

MINDFUL EATING

When was the last time you ate a meal and really focused on the meal itself? When you focus on what you are eating, your brain and body realize you are eating. Your body is more likely to produce the proper digestive enzymes for the meal, and you are more likely to feel sated. If you eat without focus, you are more likely to overeat. When you eat while driving, reading, or watching TV, food can disappear and you may not be sure what happened to it.

To eat mindfully, first pause before you eat, and breathe deeply and slowly. Take time to remember where your food comes from and to think or say a word of gratitude. This slowing down will help you enjoy your food more and will help the food to digest better. Set the table. Light a candle. Connect with someone you love. Arrange your food on a real plate and use real utensils. We feel more satisfied when we treat a meal as a worthwhile experience.

Chewing is an important first step in digestion. Enzymes in the saliva begin the process of breaking food down. Tasting the food helps get gastric juices flowing so that food can be thoroughly processed by the stomach. But this only happens if you take the time to chew well and taste your food. Chewing and tasting can make the difference between poor digestion and good digestion. Take time to savor each bite. When we pay attention to the food we are eating and really taste it, our mind registers that we have eaten, and we feel satisfied with just enough food.

Stop eating a couple of hours before you go to bed. If you are still trying to digest a heavy dinner at bedtime, you will not sleep as well and you may gain unwanted weight. Conversely, if you are starving at bedtime, it is ok to eat a bite or two so you can sleep better.

Eating with your hands is generally relegated to fast food in our society, so we have largely lost this connection with digestion. When you touch food as you are eating it, it signals the stomach to begin producing enzymes needed for digestion. Eating with your hands is a good way to eat mindfully because you tend to be more focused on food you are picking up with your fingers. It is also a good temperature gauge: you are less likely to burn your mouth if you have touched it with your fingers first.[4]

If you are at work, leave your desk for lunch and look for somewhere to eat that is a bit more inspiring. If you sit at your desk, you are likely to focus on your work or your computer, and not on the meal you are eating. If you eat while you are driving, you are not focused on your food. And chances are, you are not fully focused on your driving either, which can be dangerous.

DRINK YOUR WATER

Drinking enough water is incredibly important for your digestion. Without enough water, food does not move through your system well. How much water do you need? Here is a good rule of thumb: Take your weight in pounds, and drink half that much water each day in ounces. So a 140 pound person would need roughly 70 ounces of water. Herbal teas can be counted as part of the water you drink, but not dehydrating beverages such as coffee, tea, or sweetened drinks. The verdict is still out on drinking water with a meal. Some say that you should drink water with a meal, others believe you should drink water only between meals since water dilutes the stomach acid required to digest food. Bottom line: drink enough.

Books have been written about the types of water you should drink. There are different camps, but most people agree on these points:

- The water should be potable. Potable simply means that the water is safe to drink. Chlorine provides this function for most of us.

- The water should be free of contaminants and chemicals.

The water that is in municipal water supplies is treated to keep communities free of water-born diseases. While this is necessary, these municipalities frequently produce water that is not the best for optimum health. Chlorine is needed to kill pathogens that may be in the water, but it can be detrimental to health. In most places, you will want to filter your water. Most filters can remove chlorine. Remember to change your filter as often as the manufacturer suggests.

Fluoride in water is at the center of a greater controversy. Those in favor of fluoride say that it is of benefit for dental health. However, research has proven that fluoride added to drinking water does not benefit dental health and, in fact, can cause dental fluorosis (staining of the teeth and, in severe cases, pitting). The truth is that there is no compelling reason to add fluoride, and many health reasons why it is a bad idea. "Fluoride is an outdated form of mass-medication . . . [A] growing body of evidence reasonably indicates that fluoridated water, in addition to other sources of daily fluoride exposure, can cause or contribute to a range of serious problems, including arthritis, damage to the developing brain, reduced thyroid function, and possibly osteosarcoma (bone cancer) in adolescent males."[5] Most general filters will not remove fluoride; you must have a filter specifically for this purpose. The Fluoride Action Network is a watchdog for policies regarding fluoridation.

Try to get your water from a clean water source rather than drinking it from plastic bottles. Chemicals from the plastic can leach into the water. This is not healthy. And, producing so much plastic waste is not sustainable for our planet.

Many people object to the taste of water. Often, the objectionable taste is from chemicals. When water is filtered and pure, it has a neutral taste. If you prefer additional flavor after filtering your water, add a slice of an organic fruit or vegetable such as lemon, fresh or frozen berries, or cucumber. Suddenly, drinking water will be elevated to a mini-spa experience.

VINO DOLCE

As I was growing up, my dad, conservative though he was in almost every aspect of his life, had a hobby of making delicious country wines. As a little girl, I would sit on his lap while we watched **Lost in Space**[6] reruns together, hiding my eyes in Daddy's shirt during the scary parts. Sometimes, he had a glass of wine and would give me a sip. So I learned to appreciate wine at an early age. In this respect, our household operated in a European way—it was not forbidden for me to have a glass of wine, so long as I maintained great respect for it. Since it was not forbidden, I never felt a need to sneak or prove anything with alcohol when I arrived at my teenage years.

Some recent studies have shown that wine actually encourages the growth of gut-friendly probiotics in the stomach. Most sources agree that wine consumed in moderation, a few glasses a week, will not cause problems and may be beneficial.[7]

On the other hand, Body Ecology reports that "Researchers at the Institute of Microbiology and Wine Research at Mainz University, Germany, report that a relatively high percentage of people show signs of an intolerance to wine—specifically, red wine."[8]

Véronique Raskin of the Organic Wine Company reminds us that non-organic grapes are on the Environmental Working Group's Dirty Dozen list. "Unfortunately," says the company's website, "wine grapes receive more pesticides than table grapes."[9]

From a health standpoint, it seems that wine, consumed in moderation, especially from organic sources, can be a part of healthy eating. And, celebrating great moments with a glass of wine adds rich dimension to a life well-lived.

A SENSORY FEAST

The most basic reason to eat is to nourish our bodies. In many parts of the world, enough nourishment in any form is difficult to come by. Here in the U.S., getting enough is usually easy for most people. The problem is that many people get too much, or at least too much of foods that fill but do not nourish.

Because we have to eat to live, we have built-in cravings to encourage eating. If we eat mindlessly, just to fill up and satisfy cravings, we will not be healthy. But if we use our senses to eat (our eyes, taste, smell and touch), and choose foods that are real and whole, then eating becomes a sensory feast, filling and nourishing us. Sharing a meal and conversation with someone we care about adds to our experience and our nourishment.

As you can tell, some of my favorite memories involve food with family and friends. In recent years, our deck has become the go-to place for family gatherings in good weather. We light candles and tiki torches, throw a batik cloth on the picnic table, toss something tantalizing on the grill, whip up salads and bowls of vegetables, and open bottles of wine. Then we spend the remainder of the evening enjoying our feast, and talking and laughing into the night. My digestion always seems to work remarkably well on those occasions, as if the laughter and good company share equal importance with the nutrients in the food.

It is not always possible to eat a feast prepared for a party. But in your daily life, approach your food and your eating with joy, and give the task of nourishing your body and your soul the respect it deserves. Make your meals a sensory feast. Prepare and eat real, whole food. Treat yourself like you matter by setting a place for yourself. Pay attention to the food you eat. Take time with the process of nourishing yourself. Not enough time? Make time. Let something else in your life operate on auto-pilot, but not your food—not the stuff of life that nurtures and sustains you.

I am convinced that the future of our health depends on a return to delicious whole foods and a holistic restoration of our minds, our bodies and our spirits. Take time to eat real food. Be nourished. Be well.

recipes:

"...I finally felt bold and fearless in the kitchen, which was an entirely new feeling for me."

Aarti Sequeira

LOOKING AHEAD

Remember the menu plan we talked about in Step 2? The menus I suggested are below. The recipes follow, along with a few other simple dishes that can be used as the basis for inspired meals. All the recipes are basic because I want to give you the tools to get started. Once you are comfortable with cooking these foods, branch out and try new recipes. Look for the best possible ingredients. The simpler the recipe is, the more important the flavor of each ingredient becomes.

FIVE EASY EVERYDAY MENUS
Menu No. 1

Salade Niçoise

Just Salade Niçoise, and maybe a glass of Sauvignon blanc. There are a few steps required, but a little pre-preparation the night before, or morning of, makes this a fast, fabulous dinner. Serve it alfresco on the first warm day of summer. For fun, arrange it on a big platter and share with someone you love.

Menu No. 2

Grilled Hamburgers with Mushrooms & Salad Toppings

Quinoa Tabbouleh

Grass-fed burgers with all the trimmings. You'll never want a fast-food burger again. Add a serving of vegetable-rich Quinoa Tabbouleh that you made yesterday.

Menu No. 3

Quick Spaghetti Sauce with Spaghetti Squash

Green Salad with Vinaigrette Dressing

Quick Spaghetti is comfort food without remorse. And did I mention that it is quick? The spaghetti squash will have to be wrassled and roasted, but that is the only tricky part.

Menu No. 4

Bubbies® Chicken

Oven Roasted Cauliflower and Broccoli

Sweet Potato Salad

Make the Sweet Potato Salad ahead. The rest you can have prepared in 20 minutes, totally finished in only 30. Fast food from your kitchen.

Menu No. 5

Mediterranean Skillet with Rice

A staple at the Watson house, and really, REALLY fast. Use pastured pork sausage from your local farmer. Serve it with a simple salad or some cut up cucumbers.

GRAINS AND STARCHY VEGETABLES

These are the foods that the low-carb camp loves to hate. Your body, especially your thyroid and adrenals, need these in moderation. Make sure the "carbs" you put in your body are of the best quality and properly prepared to keep your inflammation levels low. If you want to hate carbohydrates, hate junk carbs.

Overnight Oatmeal

This recipe is an instant breakfast for crazy mornings. Oatmeal provides healthy, soluble fiber.

Ingredients:

1/2 cup of long-cooking oatmeal

1/3 - 1/2 cup of water or milk

pinch of sea salt

1 tablespoon dried fruit

nuts

fresh fruit

yogurt

Steps:

1. In a bowl, mix oatmeal, liquid and sea salt. Add dried fruit.

2. Cover and put in the fridge overnight.

3. In the morning top with nuts, fresh fruit and yogurt.

Rice

To be such a simple food, rice comes in an amazing variety of flavors. The rice that is most used in the U.S., long-grain white rice, is less flavorful than some other varieties. Short-grain rices are stickier, and are a staple in Asian cooking. For a delicious aroma, try Jasmine or Basmati rice. Wild rice is actually not a rice at all, but a grass. Since it needs to cook for about the same amount of time as brown rice, the two can be mixed. Most of the anti-nutrients are in the outer covering of brown rice. Since this covering is stripped from white rice, it does not contain as many phytates and does not need to be soaked. So, to make brown rice less inflammatory, it is important to soak it overnight. Soak wild rice as well.

Ingredients:

2 cups of rice (brown or white, or a mixture of brown and wild rices)

2 cups of filtered water for cooking, plus additional filtered water for soaking and rinsing (for unsoaked rice, make this 4 cups)

1 Tbsp vinegar, naturally fermented sauerkraut or pickle juice, or whey

Steps:

1. Rinse the grains by swirling in water, then drain through a fine mesh strainer.

2. Soak brown or wild rice. (This step can be omitted with white rice.) Pour additional filtered water over the grains to cover. Add the vinegar, sauerkraut juice, or whey. Soak overnight, or up to 24 hours to neutralize phytates.

3. Drain the brown or wild rice. Rinse it in additional filtered water. This washes away the residue from the phytates.

4. Cook. Place rice in a 2-3 quart saucepan. Add 2 cups of

filtered water (4 for unsoaked white rice). Cover the pot. Bring to a boil over medium heat. Turn the heat down and cook for an additional 14 minutes minutes for white rice, or 50 minutes for brown or wild rice. Remove the lid and fluff.

5. Enjoy rice for lunch in a bowl with fresh greens, avocado, a slice of turkey and some tamari or soy sauce. Serve as a side dish for dinner, or add to a stir-fry.

6. Store rice in the fridge for up to 5 days.

Basic Quinoa

Quinoa is my favorite grain, or more correctly, seed. It is a closer relative to beets and chard than it is to wheat and other grains. Most of the time I have quinoa at some stage of preparation in my kitchen: soaking in a jar, cooking on the stove, or stored, cooked, in the fridge, ready for a quick snack or meal.

Ingredients:

2 cups of quinoa (I mix white quinoa with small amounts of red or black quinoa for color.)

2 cups of filtered water for cooking, plus additional filtered water for soaking and rinsing

1 Tbsp vinegar, naturally fermented sauerkraut or pickle juice, or whey

Steps:

1. Rinse the grains by swirling in water, then drain through a fine mesh strainer. This gets rid of the soapy residue that is naturally present on quinoa. Many people skip this step, but the soapy residue can cause inflammation.

2. Soak the grains. Pour additional filtered water over the grains to cover. Add the vinegar, sauerkraut juice, or whey. Soak overnight, or up to 24 hours. This neutralizes about 70% of the phytates in the quinoa.

3. Drain the quinoa. Rinse it in additional filtered water. This washes away the residue from the phytates.

4. Cook. Place quinoa in a 2-3 quart saucepan. Add 2 cups of filtered water. The quinoa should be covered with water, plus an addition half-inch of water. Cover the pot. Bring to a boil over medium heat. Turn the heat down and cook for an additional 5 minutes. Keep the lid on. Turn off the heat and let the quinoa set for 10-15 minutes. Remove the lid and fluff.

5. Enjoy quinoa for breakfast with seeds and nuts, yogurt, berries and honey. Eat as a snack with a dollop of good-quality extra-virgin olive oil and a sprinkle of sea salt. Serve as a side dish for dinner, or add to a salad for extra flavor and holding power.

6. Store quinoa in the fridge for up to 5 days.

Quinoa Tabbouleh

In the summer, I make great vats of Tabbouleh and keep it in the fridge. It becomes lunch almost daily until it is gone, and makes a great side dish for supper as well. Once your quinoa has been prepared, the remaining fresh ingredients can be assembled quickly.

Ingredients:

one recipe of prepared quinoa, above

1/2 cup extra-virgin olive oil

1/4 cup lemon juice

1/4 cup apple cider vinegar

sea salt and pepper to taste

2 medium cucumbers, seeded and chopped (if the seeds of the cucumber are mature, remove them with a slice of the knife. Young, unformed seeds can be left alone.)

2 medium tomatoes seeded and chopped (seed tomatoes by raking out the seeds. Do not try to get them all - just make a quick swipe as you are cutting up the tomato.)

1 can of chick peas, rinsed and drained. (look for organic)

1 bunch of parsley, de-stemmed and chopped

1/2 cup fresh mint, chopped (this can be left out in a pinch, but it adds amazing flavor.)

Steps:

1. In a small jar, combine olive oil, lemon juice, apple cider vinegar, salt and pepper. Shake well.

2. Combine remaining ingredients, add dressing. Toss. Serve. Enjoy.

Sweet Potatoes

This is another favorite non-recipe of mine. My grandaddy used to bake sweet potatoes in the oven. In the fall and winter they were always available, ready to eat cold for a sweet and satisfying snack, or to add to other recipes for an instant soup or salad. My favorites are Garnet sweet potatoes, or Japanese white sweet potatoes. Buy organic because pesticides are used on the non-organic ones. I always choose the smaller potatoes of the lot because the big ones are sometimes stringy.

Ingredients:

6-8 sweet potatoes, more or less

butter, ghee, or olive oil

Steps:

1. Wash the potatoes well. Trim away any gnarly looking spots. Pat them dry.

2. Using the oil or butter, rub a thin coating on the potatoes. Place on a rimmed baking pan.

3. Bake at 400 degrees for 45 minutes, or until a fork stuck in the largest one shows that it is soft inside.

4. Let them cool a little, then enjoy, add to another recipe, or store in the fridge.

Sweet Potato Salad

Use Garnet sweet potatoes in this recipe for vibrant orange color and a big dose of beta carotine.

Ingredients:

3 pounds of cooked and cooled sweet potatoes (see recipe, above.)

1/4 cup canned organic roasted red peppers, diced.

the juice of 3 limes

1-2 cloves of garlic, minced

1/3 - 1/2 cup olive oil

sea salt and pepper

1/2 bunch of parsley, chopped

Steps:

1. Slice cooled potatoes into a large mixing bowl. Add red peppers and parsley.

2. In a small jar with a lid, combine lime juice, garlic, olive oil, sea salt and pepper. Shake well.

3. Pour over sweet potato mixture and toss.

Herbed Chick Peas

I usually fix these in the dead of winter. Autumn vegetables are getting old, and spring ones have not yet arrived. My tastebuds are ready for a flavorful pick-me-up, and the herbs make the house smell amazing. Herbed chick peas are more than a condiment, less than a serving of vegetables - a healthy snack. These do not require any fresh ingredients. Since I am hard core, I usually cook my chick peas from scratch. But you can also buy them in a can.

Ingredients:

1 pint of prepared chick peas

2 teaspoons dried dill weed

1/2 teaspoon sea salt

1/2 teaspoon granulated onion

1 large garlic clove, or 1/4 tsp granulated garlic

3 tablespoons olive oil

2 tablespoons apple cider vinegar

Steps:

1. Mix all ingredients except chick peas. Stir in chick peas.

2. Bake at 250 degrees for 30-45 minutes, stirring a couple of times. Cool and stir again.

3. Store in a quart glass jar in the fridge. Serve cold or warmed.

Roasted Spaghetti Squash

Spaghetti squash is readily available in markets from late August until early spring. You will need a hefty knife and a cutting board.

Ingredients:

1 large or 2 small spaghetti squashes for every 2 people

olive oil

sea salt

Steps:

1. Preheat your oven to 400 degrees.

2. Carefully cut the squash in half lengthwise. Scoop out the seeds and compost them.

3. Add a teaspoon of olive oil to a rimmed baking sheet and grease the pan with it. Lay the squash on the pan, cut side down. Add a cup of water to the baking pan.

4. Put in the preheated 400 degree oven for 40 minutes.

5. Open the oven door and see if the squash is done by poking it with a fork. If the pulp below the leathery skin seems soft, your squash is ready.

6. Remove from the oven. Flip the squashes, cut side up. Sprinkle with sea salt and olive oil, fluff with a fork. The squash will come out in tender "noodles" that look like spaghetti pasta.

7. Serve with spaghetti sauce. Or serve topped with herbs and ghee or butter.

Roasted Vegetables

Ingredients:

2-3 cups of in-season vegetables. Choose from: sweet onions, carrots, white or sweet potatoes, eggplant, asparagus, summer or winter squash, cabbage, tomatoes, sweet peas, mushrooms, celery, and sweet bell pepper (yellow, red, or green). Or add your favorite vegetable.

1-2 tablespoons liquid seasoning. Choose from: balsamic vinegar (sweet, vinegary), umiboshi plum sauce (a salty Asian vinegar), sriracha sauce (hot!) or soy sauce (sweet-salty)

1-3 teaspoons dry seasoning. Choose from: paprika, pepper, basil, garlic powder, onion powder

sea salt

2-3 tablespoons olive oil

Steps:

1. Preheat oven to 400 degrees.

2. Cut up vegetables into large bite-size pieces.

3. Add a tablespoon or two of liquid seasoning. Add dry seasoning liberally - it is hard to get too much. Add a sprinkle of sea salt and the olive oil.

4. Toss ingredients together and place in the preheated oven for 20 minutes.

5. Stir the vegetables, roast 20 minutes more until the vegetables are browned and tender.

FRUITS AND NON-STARCHY VEGETABLES

Lavish your plate with vegetables of every color. Add a few fruits and you will have a cornucopia of nutrient rich foods.

Green Salad with Vinaigrette Dressing

Choose fresh, organic ingredients for a memorable salad

Ingredients:

lettuce—choose from Romaine lettuce, Butter Crunch lettuce, or mixed salad greens.

cherry tomatoes

green onions

carrots

celery

Steps:

1. Wash all ingredients and drain thoroughly.

2. Use a potato peeler to make large slices of carrots. Slice green onions and celery. Break lettuce, unless using a salad mix.

3. Toss salad ingredients together with vinaigrette dressing.

Sunshine Vinaigrette Dressing

Ingredients:

4 tablespoons lemon juice

1 tablespoon dijon mustard

1/2 cup extra virgin olive oil

sea salt and pepper to taste

Optional: 2 tsp raw honey or to taste

Optional: 1/4 teaspoon turmeric (immune boosting, and gives a
   bright yellow color)

Steps:

1. Combine ingredients in a small jar with a tight lid and shake
    well.

Pan-fried Zucchini with Capers and Dill

Look for organic zucchini if possible.

Ingredients:

3 small to medium zucchini

1 tablespoon avocado oil or ghee

1/2 - 1 teaspoon dried dill weed

1-2 tablespoons capers

sea salt

Steps:

1. Cut zucchini in half lengthwise, then in to half-circles.

2. Heat avocado oil or ghee in a heavy skillet. When the oil is hot enough to sizzle a drop of water, add zucchini to the skillet. Stir frequently until it begins to brown and become crisp-tender.

3. Add 1/2 to 1 teaspoon of dill, a sprinkle of sea salt, and a couple of tablespoons of capers. Toss and serve.

Pan-fried Bell Peppers and Onions

Bell peppers are on the Environmental Working Group's Dirty Dozen list because of high levels of pesticides. Look for organic or grow your own. To grow: Plant in late spring or early summer. Water every few days when it doesn't rain, and wait. And wait. In the autumn you will suddenly have a bumper crop. Sweet onions are labeled in the grocery store as "sweet" or "Vidalia."

Ingredients:

1 green bell pepper

1 red bell pepper

1 yellow bell pepper

1 large sweet onion

1 teaspoon dried thyme

sea salt

Steps:

1. Slice bell peppers and sweet onion into lengthwise strips.

2. Heat avocado oil over medium high heat in a large, heavy skillet.

3. Add the onion and stir-fry until onion begins to cook. Add vegetables gradually, stirring. (You are adding gradually to keep the skillet from cooling down.)

4. Add thyme and a sprinkle of sea salt.

5. Continue stirring until vegetables are crisp-tender and intensely colorful. Serve immediately.

Super-flavorful variation: Instead of avocado oil or ghee, cook one slice of pasture-raised bacon in the skillet until it is crispy. Remove bacon. Continue with the recipe, using the bacon fat. At the end, crumble the piece of bacon into the skillet and stir before serving.

Sautéed Mushrooms

Serve over burgers.

Ingredients:

1 pound mushrooms of your choice - button, shitake, portobello, cremini or a mixture

3 tablespoons butter or ghee (more or less)

sea salt and pepper

a splash of wine

Steps:

1. Clean mushrooms by wiping them off with a damp cloth. Remove the stems. Slice into thick slices.

2. In a heavy skillet, melt a liberal amount of butter or ghee. When the butter is hot, begin adding the mushrooms. Stir and turn, keeping the temperature hot enough to sizzle.

3. After all the butter or ghee is absorbed, you may want to add a lid to the skillet just for a couple of minutes and then remove the lid and continue to stir. What you are aiming for is a skillet that is continually sizzling, but has enough moisture and fat to cook the mushrooms.

4. When they are done (this is subjective - cook a little or brown a lot) remove from the heat and add salt and pepper to taste.

5. Optionally you can add a slosh of wine while the mushrooms are still sizzling in the skillet at the end of the cooking time.

Soffrito

Soffrito, from Italy, is quick, sustaining comfort food. Years ago I bought the cookbook **Bringing Tuscany Home**[1], by Frances Mayes, author of **Under the Tuscan Sun**[2]. I have been cooking soffrito ever since then. This recipe was adapted from hers.

Ingredients:

2 large carrots

2 stalks of celery

1 medium-sized yellow onion

3-4 tablespoons olive oil

1/2 bunch of parsley

sea salt

Steps:

1. Chop the carrots, onions, and celery separately until they are about the size of corn niblets.

2. Chop the parsley finely and set aside. You should have about 1/4 cup of chopped parsley.

3. Warm a heavy skillet on the stove over medium heat until a drop of added water sizzles. Add the olive oil and swirl it around. (Be brave and do not measure it.)

4. Add the chopped onion, stirring continuously until the onion just begins to turn translucent, about 4-5 minutes. Keep the temperature high enough that it continues to sizzle.

5. Add the carrots and continue stirring until the carrot begins to soften, about 3-4 minutes.

6. Add the celery and continue stirring until the onion is cooked, the carrot is tender, and the celery is crisp - cooked.

7. Remove from the heat. Add the parsley and a sprinkle of sea salt. Toss and serve.

Roasted Tomatoes

Roasted tomatoes are favorite fare at my house. I take them along (along with soffrito) any time I am asked to bring a dish. Saturday mornings are a good time to bake these, when you are around the house, but doing other things. Use organic tomatoes for better flavor and nutrition. This recipe was also inspired by the book *Bringing Tuscany Home*.

Ingredients:

3 (28 oz.) cans of whole tomatoes

1 tablespoon dried rosemary

1 tablespoon dried oregano

1 tablespoon dried thyme

1 tablespoon dried basil

1/4 - 1/2 cup of olive oil

6 cloves of minced garlic

sea salt and pepper

Steps:

1. Preheat oven to 200 degrees F.

2. Open cans of tomatoes and drain. Save the liquid for another recipe. Cut each tomato in half lengthwise, and arrange on an oiled, rimmed baking pan. Three cans will fill a baking sheet that is about 12" x 17". There will be some liquid in the pan with the tomatoes.

3. Sprinkle the minced garlic over the tomatoes, and then the herbs. Sprinkle with sea salt and pepper. Top with the olive oil.

4. Rub a large tablespoon over the tomatoes and herbs until all of the herbs are moistened from the tomato juice and olive oil.

5. Bake for 2 hours. Your house will smell marvelous.

6. Remove from the oven and enjoy.

7. Store in the fridge in a quart glass jar for up to a week.

8. Store extra in the fridge and reheat in a skillet when you want fast food.

Roasted Broccoli and Cauliflower

Ingredients:

1 bunch of fresh broccoli

1 head of cauliflower

1/4 - 1/3 cup avocado oil or olive oil

sea salt and pepper

granulated garlic and granulated onion

coarse ground mustard

Steps:

1. Preheat oven to 500 degrees.

2. Slice broccoli and cauliflower into large-bite sized pieces.

3. In a large mixing bowl, toss with olive oil and plenty of sea salt and pepper. Optionally, sprinkle with granulated garlic and granulated onion powder.

4. Place on a rimmed baking sheet. Bake for 12 minutes until the tops begin to brown. That is all!

5. Serve with mustard. Yes, mustard tastes amazing.

Vegetables from the Freezer

Yes, I know. You have fixed these before. But people often complain about the taste of frozen vegetables. The way you prepare them can make a vast difference in flavor. I add frozen vegetables to a lot of my other recipes. But this recipe is a fool-proof method to get some tasty vegetables ready for dinner in a hurry. Use organic vegetables—they taste better and are better for you.

Ingredients:

1 package of frozen vegetables, your choice.

filtered water

1-2 tablespoons olive oil (or other healthy oil)

sea salt

1 teaspoon thyme or rosemary

Steps:

1. Remove vegetables from the freezer just before you cook them. If you thaw them first, they will taste "off." Put your vegetables in a sauce pan that has a cover.

2. Add enough water to cover the bottom by 1/2 inch.

3. Add the olive oil. The oil will improve the texture and taste of the vegetables. Some vegetables stay stringy without the addition of the oil.

4. Add herbs; rosemary to green beans, or thyme to other vegetables. Sprinkle with sea salt.

5. Cover and bring to a simmer over medium heat. When it begins steaming turn down the eye to the lowest setting. Use low heat to keep the pot from boiling dry. If you find that your stove is cooking off the liquid before the vegetables are done, add a little more.

6. Cook until done. "Done" means different things for different vegetables. For green beans, it may take 30 minutes - you want them to be soft and a dull green. Green peas are ready about 3 minutes after they begin steaming. For other vegetables, they are done when they are soft enough to suit your taste. Cook them until they lose the intense green color, but not enough for them to be mashed and soggy. Remember that the longer you cook a vegetable, the more nutrients it loses.

7. Taste. Add additional olive oil, or add a pat of butter and a bit more sea salt if needed for the best flavor.

MEATS AND MAIN DISHES

Salad Niçoise

Recipes for this French classic salad abound on the internet. Probably the most famous version comes from Julia Child's book **The Way To Cook**[2]. Salade Niçoise, to me, is the perfect summer meal—beautiful, fresh, and tasty. My inspiration for this recipe comes from Martha Stewart Living's Cookbook, **Everyday Food: Great Food Fast**[3]. In the summer we have this salad weekly, and vary the ingredients according to what is in season and what fish we find to cook.

Ingredients:

1/2 pound new potatoes (organic, please) cut into 1-2 inch pieces

1/2 pound new, thin green beans, trimmed OR one bunch of asparagus, trimmed

1 pound salmon or tuna steaks, or you can use a can of sustainably caught yellow-fin tuna packed in olive oil. (This kind of tuna has less mercury than regular tuna.)

1 large or 2 small heads of Romaine lettuce

4 fresh tomatoes, cut into wedges and de-seeded

3 pasture-raised eggs, boiled, cooled and sliced into wedges

1 small red onion, sliced thinly

1 jar or tin of anchovy fillets, drained (do not skip this - it is yummy.)

1/4 cup pitted olives

Dijon Vinaigrette

2 tablespoons fresh lemon juice

1 tablespoon Dijon mustard

sea salt and pepper

1/4 cup olive oil

Steps:

1. In a large saucepan, add potatoes. Add 1/2 inch of filtered water. Cover, bring to a boil over medium heat, reduce to simmer. Cook 7-8 minutes. Add green beans and/or asparagus. Cover and continue cooking until green beans are crisp tender and potatoes are done. Drain and set aside on a plate to cool.

2. (Skip this step if using canned tuna.) In the same large sauce pan, add 1/4 inch of water and bring to a boil. Meanwhile, salt and pepper your fish. Lower the fish into the boiling water. Cover and cook for 10-12 minutes, until the fish is opaque.

3. Arrange salad greens in a large bowl or on a tray. Top with tomatoes, onions, eggs, anchovies, and olives. Add potatoes, green beans, and/or asparagus.

4. Combine all the ingredients of the dressing in a small jar with a tight lid. Shake well and pour over the whole salad.

Grass-fed Hamburger Patties

I buy grass-fed beef on sale, then make up several pounds of hamburger patties and freeze them on waxed paper on a cookie sheet. A day later I remove them from the cookie sheet and store in a freezer container. When I want fast food, I remove some patties from the freezer and cook them.

Ingredients:

1 pound grass-fed beef

1 tablespoon dijon mustard (or whatever mustard you like)

1 tablespoon wheat-free tamari sauce (or you could use Worcestershire sauce)

1 teaspoon oregano or rosemary (optional, but good.)

Steps:

1. Mix ingredients together, and form into 3 large or 4 smaller hamburger patties.

2. Optional: freeze.

3. Optional: remove from freezer. While patties are still frozen, put them in a cool skillet. Cover and turn the skillet on medium low. When steam begins to escape from the skillet, take off the lid.

4. Heat the skillet to medium or a little higher. Hamburger should sizzle as it is cooking. Cook until burger is done the amount you like it. If you cook it well-done, it may be tough since grass-fed beef is naturally lean.

5. A note about grass-fed beef: My grass-fed beef has a good amount of healthy, omega-3 rich fat mixed in and it fries very well without added oils or fats. Yours may be incredibly lean. If it is too lean to fry, you may want to seek out another source for your grass-fed beef. If it is a little lean, you can use a bit of coconut oil, olive oil, or ghee in your skillet to keep it from sticking.

Quick Spaghetti Sauce

Ingredients:

2 pounds grass-fed ground beef

2 diced yellow onions

2 cloves of garlic, minced, chopped or smashed

2 teaspoons oregano

2 teaspoons sea salt

2 teaspoons chili powder

2 small bay leaves or one large

2 dashes of tabasco

1 (28 oz.) can of chunky tomato sauce (organic, please)

1 (15 oz.) can tomato sauce (ditto organic)

Steps:

1. Brown grass-fed ground beef in a heavy skillet, adding additional olive oil or coconut oil if it is too lean to brown.

2. Remove browned beef to a plate. In the same skillet, brown the yellow onions.

3. Add all ingredients, bring to a simmer, cook on low heat until well done, 30 minutes.

4. Discard bay leaves. Serve over Roasted Spaghetti Squash

Bubbies® Chicken

Bubbies® Chicken is my favorite fast food. I love Bubbies® because their pickles and sauerkraut taste amazing and are fermented. This means that they are loaded with health-giving probiotic bacteria. In this recipe, you do not get the probiotics because the pickles are cooked, but you get loads of flavor and the ease of fast preparation.

Ingredients:

1 package boneless chicken thighs

ghee, coconut oil or butter for browning chicken thighs

sea salt, pepper

paprika or smoked paprika

2 Bubbies® Pickles

1/4 cup of the juice from Bubbies Pickles

Steps:

1. Cut each chicken thigh into 3 pieces.

2. In a heavy skillet, heat the oil until it sizzles when a drop of water is added. Add chicken thighs a few at a time and brown. They do not have to be completely done, just surface browned. Remove chicken thighs to a clean plate and continue frying the remaining pieces until all of the chicken pieces are browned

3. Meanwhile, chop two pickles.

4. Return all chicken pieces to the skillet. Sprinkle pickles over the top, and add juice to the skillet. Sprinkle paprika heavily over the chicken, and sprinkle with sea salt and pepper.

5. Cover skillet and simmer 5-10 minutes until chicken is cooked. Remove the lid and let remaining liquid boil away until a small amount of a thick sauce remains. Serve.

Mediterranean Skillet with Rice

Fast food at its best. You have your rice soaking (you do, no?) Use the Rice recipe above to get it cooking, then begin making the Mediterranean Skillet recipe.

Ingredients:

1 pound breakfast sausage from pasture-raised pork

1 small onion, diced

2-3 small zucchini, diced. You want 2-3 cups of zucchini

1/2 cup green pepper, diced

1 clove of garlic, minced or chopped

1 teaspoon oregano

1 (8 oz.) can of tomato sauce

Steps:

1. In a heavy skillet, brown sausage and onion. Pour off excess fat.

2. Add remaining ingredients and stir.

3. Cover and cook about 15 minutes until zucchini is done. Serve with cooked rice, see recipe above.

Super fast:

Instead of fixing rice separately, you can also add 1/3 cup of white rice and 1/2 cup of water to this recipe when you add the zucchini. Cover and cook until all the liquid is absorbed and the rice is done. (But I like my rice best cooked separately.)

A note about skillets:

A heavy iron or carbon steel skillet is best for browning. However, you do not want to cook liquids in general, or tomatoes in particular, in an unfinished iron skillet. If you are cooking in an enameled skillet, follow this recipe exactly. Otherwise, you may want to brown your meat and cook this dish in a sauce pan, or transfer the skillet-cooked meat to a sauce pan before adding other ingredients. Cooking liquids, and especially tomatoes, in iron leaches too many metals into the dish.

CONDIMENTS

Herbes de Provence

I spent some time in France with my daughter and went on a driving tour to explore the country. In Arles, after dining next door to the place where Van Gogh painted *Café Terrace at Night*, I bought Herbes de Provence from a vendor. I used these herbs to cook throughout the remainder of my journey and saved the label, which had the ingredients: *romarin, thym, basilic, marjolaine, sarriette.* Here is the recipe I invented when I got home to remind me of the taste of France. Every year when I am yearning for spring I make several recipes and put Herbes de Provence on almost everything I cook. Find the herbs at your local natural grocery. Mix together and store in a small glass jar:

Ingredients:

4 teaspoons crushed dried rosemary

4 teaspoons thyme

4 teaspoons basil

2 teaspoons marjoram

2 teaspoons oregano

2 teaspoons savory

Ghee

Ghee, also called clarified butter, is what is left when the milk solids are removed from butter. It can be stored at room temperature, and can be eaten by most people even if they are sensitive to dairy. Because the milk solids have been removed, ghee has a higher smoke point and can be used for frying. Ghee has a lot of health benefits, especially for the digestive system. It is easy to make.

Ingredients:

1 pound of unsalted butter

Steps:

1. Bring butter to a boil in a saucepan over medium heat.

2. Let it simmer in an open pan until the milk solids either rise to the top or fall to the bottom. Sometimes both can happen. This generally happens within a minute or two after the butter comes to a boil. If you want your ghee to have the traditional browned flavor of Indian ghee, let it continue to cook until the milk solids begin to brown.

3. Remove from the stovetop, then skim any milk solids off the top. Pour the remaining golden liquid into a canning jar. Stop pouring when the milk solids at the bottom begin to be poured.

4. Discard the milk solids and let the ghee cool. Store at room temperature.

Note: I make at least two pounds at a time.

REFERENCES

Introduction
[1] *The Hobbit: An Unexpected Journey.* Dir. Peter Jackson. Perf. Ian McKellen, Martin Freeman, Richard Armitage. Warner Brothers UK, 2013. DVD.

Step 1: Return to Real Foods
[1] Bianco, Margery Williams. *The Velveteen Rabbit, Or, How Toys Become Real.* New York: Holt, Rinehart and Winston, 1983. Print.

[2] *Super Size Me.* Dir. Morgan Spurlock. Perf. Morgan Spurlock. Cameo, 2005. DVD.

[3] Sisson, Mark. "The 80/20 Principle: When 20 Inches Toward 40 | Mark's Daily Apple." *Marks Daily Apple RSS.* Mark Sisson, 21 Apr. 2010. Web. 11 Mar. 2015. <http://www.marksdailyapple.com/the-80-20-principle-when-20-inches-toward-40/#axzz3U5eQjaO7>.

[4] Dwyer, Marge. "Eating Healthy vs. Unhealthy Diet Costs about $1.50 More per Day." Harvard T.H. *Chan School of Public Health.* The President and Fellows of Harvard College, 5 Dec. 2013. Web. 27 Feb. 2015. <http%3A%2F%2Fwww.hsph.harvard.edu%2Fnews%2Fpress-releases%2Fhealthy-vs-unhealthy-diet-costs-1-50-more%2F>.

[5] Pollan, Michael. *In Defense of Food: An Eater's Manifesto.* New York: Penguin, 2008. 187-188. Print.

Step 2: Devise a (Grocery) Market Strategy
(no references)

Step 3: Stock your pantry
[1] "Cotton." Cotton. N.p., n.d. Web. 24 Feb. 2015. <http://www.panna.org/resources/cotton>.

[2] "Color Additive Status List." Color Additive Status List. N.p., n.d. Web. 24 Feb. 2015. <http://www.fda.gov/ForIndustry/ColorAdditives/ColorAdditiveInventories/ucm106626.htm>.

[3] "Foods Americans Eat That Are Banned around the World." Fox News. FOX News Network, 23 Oct. 2013. Web. 24 Feb. 2015. <http://www.foxnews.com/leisure/2013/10/23/10-foods-americans-eat-that-are-banned-around-world/>.

[4] "What Is the Meaning of 'natural' on the Label of Food?" What Is the Meaning of 'natural' on the Label of Food? N.p., n.d. Web. 20 Feb. 2015. <http://www.fda.gov/aboutfda/transparency/basics/ucm214868.htm>.

[5] Spector, Dina. "The Surprising Truth About How Many Chemicals Are In Everything

We Eat." Business Insider. Business Insider, Inc, 03 Feb. 2014. Web. 24 Feb. 2015. <http://www.businessinsider.com/facts-about-natural-and-artificial-flavors-2014-1>.

[6] Blaylock, Russell L. "Introduction." *Excitotoxins: The Taste That Kills*. Santa Fe, NM: Health, 1998. Xvii-ix. Print.

[7] Davis, William. *Wheat Belly: Lose the Wheat, Lose the Weight, and Find Your Path Back to Health*. Emmaus, Penn.: Rodale, 2011. Print.

[8] "The Truth About Saturated Fats and The Coconut Oil Benefits." *Mercola.com*. Joseph Mercola, 22 Oct. 2010. Web. 11 Mar. 2015. <http://articles.mercola.com/sites/articles/archive/2010/10/22/coconut-oil-and-saturated-fats-can-make-you-healthy.aspx>.

Step 4: Get Your Fruits and Veggies

[1] *VeggieTales Greatest Hits*. Big Idea Records, 2008. CD.

[2] "The Ultimate Guide to Antioxidants." *Mercola.com*. N.p., n.d. Web. 26 Feb. 2015. <http://articles.mercola.com/antioxidants.aspx>.

[3] Drake, Karen S. "Natural Sun Protection." *Dr Frank Lipman*. Dr. Frank Lipman, 22 July 2011. Web. 14 Mar. 2015. <http://www.drfranklipman.com/natural-sun-protection/>.

[4] "Food Miles: How Far Your Food Travels Has Serious Consequences for Your Health and the Climate." **Health Facts** (n.d.): n. pag. Nov. 2007. Web. 2 Mar. 2015. <https://food-hub.org/files/resources/Food%20Miles.pdf>.

[5] "Fixing the Oversight of Chemicals Added to Our Food." *Pew Trusts*. The Pew Charitable Trusts, 7 Nov. 2013. Web. 15 Mar. 2015. <http://www.pewtrusts.org/en/research-and-analysis/reports/2013/11/07/fixing-the-oversight-of-chemicals-added-to-our-food>.

[6] "USDA Claims Pesticide Residues in Food Is Safe." *Mercola.com*. N.p., n.d. Web. 26 Feb. 2015. <http://articles.mercola.com/sites/articles/archive/2015/01/27/glyphosate-gmo-pesticide-residue.aspx>.

[7] "National Organic Program." *Agricultural Marketing Service*. N.p., n.d. Web. 27 Feb. 2015. <http://www.ams.usda.gov/AMSv1.0/NOPOrganicStandards>.

[8] "EWG's Shopper's Guide to Pesticides in Produce™." *Environmental Working Group*. N.p., n.d. Web. 01 Mar. 2015. <http://www.ewg.org/foodnews/list.php>.

[9] "Radiation Protection - Food Safety." *EPA*. Environmental Protection Agency, n.d. Web. 25 Feb. 2015. <http://www.epa.gov/radiation/sources/food_safety.html>.

[10] "What's Wrong with Food Irradiation?" *Organic Consumers Association*. N.p., n.d. Web. 26 Feb. 2015. <https://www.organicconsumers.org/old_articles/Irrad/irradfact.php>.

[11] "Food Irradiation." *EPA*. Environmental Protection Agency, n.d. Web. 01 Mar. 2015. <http://www3.epa.gov/radtown/food-irradiation.html>.

[12] "Frequently Asked Questions on Genetically Modified Foods." *WHO*. World Health Organization, n.d. Web. 11 Feb. 2015. <http://www.who.int/foodsafety/areas_work/food-technology/faq-genetically-modified-food/en/>.

[13] Smith, Jeffrey M. "Genetically Modified Corn Study Reveals Health Damage and Cover-up." *Institute for Responsible Technology*. N.p., 2005. Web. 01 Mar. 2015. <http://www.responsibletechnology.org/fraud/rigged-studies/Genetically-Modified-Corn-Study-Reveals-Health-Damage-and-Cover-up-June-2005>.

[14] "The Non-GMO Project." *The NonGMO Project*. N.p., n.d. Web. 26 Feb. 2015. <http://www.nongmoproject.org/>.

Step 5: Stock the Larder

[1] Pollan, Michael. *In Defense of Food: An Eater's Manifesto*. New York: Penguin, 2008. Print.

[2] "Nutritional Typing Diet - Know Your Nutritional Type and Modify Your Diet so You Feel Terrific." *Mercola.com*. N.p., n.d. Web. 02 Mar. 2015. <http://articles.mercola.com/sites/articles/archive/2003/02/26/metabolic-typing-part-three.aspx>.

[3] Freund, Daisy. "How Animal Welfare Leads to Better Meat: A Lesson From Spain." *The Atlantic*. Atlantic Media Company, 25 Aug. 2011. Web. 02 Mar. 2015. <http://www.theatlantic.com/health/archive/2011/08/how-animal-welfare-leads-to-better-meat-a-lesson-from-spain/244127/>.

[4] Kirby, David. Introduction. *Animal Factory: The Looming Threat of Industrial Pig, Dairy, and Poultry Farms to Humans and the Environment*. New York: St. Martin's Griffin, 2011. xii. Print.

[5] Kirby, xiv

[6] Robbins, John. "The Truth About Grassfed Beef." *Food Revolution Network*. John and Ocean Robbins, 19 Dec. 2012. Web. 07 Mar. 2015. <http://foodrevolution.org/blog/the-truth-about-grassfed-beef/>.

[7] "Pigs - the Farm Connoisseurs of the Farm Animal Kingdom." *Natural Pig Farming.* N.p., 2013. Web. 7 Mar. 2015. <http%3A%2F%2Fwww.naturalpigfarming.com%2Ffeed. htm>.

[8] Achitoff-Gray, Niki. "Cooking Fats 101: What's a Smoke Point and Why Does It Matter?" *Serious Eats.* N.p., 16 May 2014. Web. 18 Mar. 2015. <http://www.seriouseats. com/2014/05/cooking-fats-101-whats-a-smoke-point-and-why-does-it-matter.html>.

[9] Cheng, Vivian, RHN. "What Is Margarine and Why Is It Bad for You? - The Real Food Guide." *The Real Food Guide.* Vivian Cheng, 13 June 2013. Web. 07 Mar. 2015. <http:// therealfoodguide.com/what-is-margarine-and-why-is-it-bad-for-you/>.

[10] Fallon, Sally, and Mary G. Enig, PhD. "The Skinny on Fats." *Weston A Price.* N.p., 1 Jan. 2000. Web. 07 Mar. 2015. <http://www.westonaprice.org/health-topics/ the-skinny-on-fats/#2>.

[11] Mercola, Joseph, D.O. "The Cholesterol Myth That Could Be Harming Your Health." *The Huffington Post.* TheHuffingtonPost.com, 12 Aug. 2010. Web. 07 Mar. 2015. <http:// www.huffingtonpost.com/dr-mercola/the-cholesterol-myth-that_b_676817.html>.

[12] Benfit, Emily. "Think Fat-Free Milk Is Healthy? 6 Secrets You Don't Know About Skim." *Butter Believer.* Emily Benfit, n.d. Web. 08 Mar. 2015. <http://butterbeliever.com/ fat-free-dairy-skim-milk-secrets/>.

[13] Houghton, Lisa A., and Reinhold Vieth. "The Case against Ergocalciferol (vitamin D2) as a Vitamin Supplement." *The American Journal of Clinical Nutrition.* American Society for Clinical Nutrition, 5 May 2006. Web. 22 Mar. 2015. <http://ajcn.nutrition. org/content/84/4/694.full>.

[14] Wiess, Kenneth R. "Fish Farms Become Feedlots of the Sea." *Los Angeles Times.* Los Angeles Times, 9 Dec. 2002. Web. 08 Mar. 2015. <http://www.latimes.com/nation/la- me-salmon9dec09-story.html#page=1>.

[15] Sisson, Mark. "Factory Farmed vs Wild Salmon | Mark's Daily Apple." *Marks Daily Apple.* N.p., 12 Sept. 2008. Web. 08 Mar. 2015. <http://www.marksdailyapple.com/ salmon-factory-farm-vs-wild/#axzz3Toz0Td1L>.

[16] Wright, Brierly, M.S, R.D. "6 of the Healthiest Fish to Eat (and 6 to Avoid)." *Eating Well.* N.p., 22 Feb. 2012. Web. 08 Mar. 2015. <http://www.eatingwell.com/blogs/ health_blog/6_of_the_healthiest_fish_to_eat_and_6_to_avoid>.

[17] Weil, Andrew, M.D. "Q & A Library: Avoid Tilapia?" *Dr. Weil.* N.p., 28 Oct. 2008. Web. 08 Mar. 2015. <http://www.drweil.com/drw/u/QAA400472/Avoid-Tilapia.html>.

Step 6: Have Your Just Desserts

[1] Aronson, Marc, and Marina Tamar. Budhos. "From Magic to Spice." *Sugar Changed the World: A Story of Magic, Spice, Slavery, Freedom, and Science*. Boston: Clarion, 2010. 9-29. Print.

[2] Casey, John. "The Hidden Ingredient That Can Sabotage Your Diet." *WebMD*. WebMD, 3 Jan. 2005. Web. 10 Mar. 2015. <http://www.webmd.com/diet/the-hidden-ingredient-that-can-sabotage-your-diet>.

[3] Upton, Julie, RD. "New Sugar Guidelines: Not-So-Sweet News for Your Heart." *Health News / Tips & Trends / Celebrity Health*. Health Media Ventures, Inc., 10 Sept. 2009. Web. 10 Mar. 2015. <http://news.health.com/2009/09/10/new-sugar-guidelines-not-so-sweet-news-for-your-heart/>.

[4] Appleton, Nancy, PhD. "141 Reasons Sugar Ruins Your Health." *Nancy Appleton Books Health Blog*. N.p., 14 June 2010. Web. 12 Mar. 2015. <http://nancyappleton.com/141-reasons-sugar-ruins-your-health/>.

[5] Laskawy, Tom. "What a 'Sweet Surprise'! HFCS Contains More Fructose than Believed." *Grist.org*. Grist, 26 Oct. 2010. Web. 12 Mar. 2015. <http://grist.org/article/food-2010-10-26-hfcs-contains-more-fructose-than-claimed/>.

[6] Hyman, Mark, M.D. "5 Reasons High Fructose Corn Syrup Will Kill You." *Dr Mark Hyman*. N.p., 13 May 2011. Web. 09 Mar. 2015. <http://drhyman.com/blog/2011/05/13/5-reasons-high-fructose-corn-syrup-will-kill-you/>.

[7] "Artificial Sweeteners and Cancer." *National Cancer Institute*. N.p., n.d. Web. 12 Mar. 2015. <http://www.cancer.gov/cancertopics/causes-prevention/risk-factors/diet/artificial-sweeteners-fact-sheet>.

[8] Schernhammer, E. S. "Consumption of Artificial Sweetener- and Sugar-containing Soda and Risk of Lymphoma and Leukemia in Men and Women." *National Center for Biotechnology Information*. U.S. National Library of Medicine, 24 Oct. 2012. Web. 12 Mar. 2015. <http://www.ncbi.nlm.nih.gov/pubmed/23097267>.

[9] Suez, Jotham, et al. "Artificial Sweeteners Induce Glucose Intolerance by Altering the Gut Microbiota." *Nature.com*. Nature Publishing Group, 9 Oct. 2014. Web. 12 Mar. 2015. <http://www.nature.com/articles/nature13793.html>.

[10] Cong, Wei-na. "Long-Term Artificial Sweetener Acesulfame Potassium Treatment Alters Neurometabolic Functions in C57BL/6J Mice." *PLOS ONE:*. N.p., 7 Aug. 2013. Web. 22 Mar. 2015. <http://journals.plos.org/plosone/article?id=10.1371%2Fjournal.pone.0070257>.

[11] Nordqvist, Joseph. "What Are the Health Benefits of Honey?" *Medical News Today*. MediLexicon International, 26 Sept. 2014. Web. 12 Mar. 2015. <http://www.medicalnewstoday.com/articles/264667.php>.

[12] Pollan, Michael, and Maira Kalman. "#45." *Food Rules: An Eater's Manual*. New York: Penguin, 2011. 126. Print.

Step 7: Prepare Simple Fare

[1] Chaplin, Amy. *At Home in the Whole Food Kitchen: Celebrating the Art of Eating Well*. Boston: Shambhala Publications, 2014. Print.

[2] Martha Stewart Living Magazine. *Everyday Food: Great Food Fast*. New York: Clarkson Potter, 2007. Print.

[3] Mayfield, Julie, and Charles Mayfield. *Paleo Comfort Foods: Homestyle Cooking for a Gluten-free Kitchen*. Las Vegas, NV: Victory Belt Pub., 2011. Print.

[4] Bittman, Mark. *Mark Bittman's Kitchen Express: 404 Inspired Seasonal Dishes You Can Make in 20 Minutes or Less*. New York: Simon & Schuster, 2009. Print.

[5] Miller, Magnolia. "What Are Xenoestrogens and How Do They Make You Fat?" *What Are Xenoestrogens and How Do They Make You Fat?* Healthline Networks, Inc., 21 June 2012. Web. 13 Mar. 2015. <http://www.healthline.com/health-blogs/hold-that-pause/what-are-xenoestrogens-fat>.

[6] Zeratsky, Katherine, R.D., L.D. "What Is BPA, and What Are the Concerns about BPA?" *Healthy Lifestyle - Nutrition and Healthy Eating*. Mayo Clinic, 21 May 2013. Web. 21 Mar. 2015. <http://www.mayoclinic.org/healthy-living/nutrition-and-healthy-eating/expert-answers/bpa/faq-20058331>.

Step 8: Eat Well

[1] *Captain Ron--electronic Press Kit*. Dir. Daryn Okada and Thom Eberhardt. Perf. Kurt Russell, Marvin Short and Mary Kay Place. Buena Vista Home Entertainment, 1992. DVD.

[2] "The Importance of Family Dinners VIII." *CASAColumbia*. The National Center on Addiction and Substance Abuse at Columbia University, Sept. 2012. Web. 15 Mar. 2015. <http://www.casacolumbia.org/addiction-research/reports/importance-of-family-dinners-2012>.

[3] Thacker, Darshana. "Food With Prana: 12 Principles of Ayurvedic Food | The Mindful Word." *The Mindful Word*. N.p., 16 Jan. 2013. Web. 15 Mar. 2015. <http://www.themindfulword.org/2013/ayurvedic-food-principles/>.

[4] Sampath, Pavitra. "Why Eating with Your Hands Is Good for Health." *The Health Site*. India Webportal Private Limited, 7 Aug. 2014. Web. 15 Mar. 2015. <http://www.thehealthsite.com/diseases-conditions/why-eating-with-your-hands-is-good-for-health/>.

[5] "Water Fluoridation." *Fluoridealert.org*. Fluoride Action Network, n.d. Web. 20 Mar. 2015. <http://fluoridealert.org/issues/water/>.

[6] Allen, Irwin, prod. *Lost in Space*. 1965. Television.

[7] Cohen, Hiyaguha. "Red Wine Helps the Gut." *Increased Digestive Probiotics Among Benefits of Red Wine*. Jon Barron, Baseline of Health Foundation, 22 May 2012. Web. 15 Mar. 2015. <http://jonbarron.org/article/red-wine-helps-gut#.VKN9h1rwZBU>.

[8] "Does Red Wine Cause Inflammation In the Gut? / All Body Ecology Articles." *Body Ecology*. Body Ecology, 15 Jan. 2014. Web. 15 Mar. 2015. <http://bodyecology.com/articles/does-red-wine-cause-inflammation-in-the-gut#.VQXzFzplhBU>.

[9] Raskin, Véronique. "FAQs - What Is Organic Wine? | The Organic Wine Company." *The Organic Wine Company*. The Organic Wine Company, n.d. Web. 15 Mar. 2015. <http://theorganicwinecompany.com/faqs/#q4>.

Recipes:

[1] Mayes, Frances. *Bringing Tuscany Home: Sensuous Style from the Heart of Italy*. New York: Broadway, 2004. Print.

[2] Child, Julia. *The Way to Cook*. New York: Knopf, 1993. Print.

[3] Martha Stewart Living Magazine. "Spring." *Everyday Food: Great Food Fast*. New York: Clarkson Potter, 2007. 66. Print.

About the Author:

Camille Watson began her lifelong study of nutrition and healthy living over thirty years ago as she earned her degree in Nutrition. Her personal health adventures with celiac, food allergies and digestion made her realize the value of having an informed advocate, and has given her a heart for helping others navigate the sometimes confusing maze of information. Today she teaches individuals and groups how to restore their own health through delicious whole foods and lifestyle transformations.

Camille serves clients as a one-on-one coach, a speaker, a teacher, and an author. Her philosophy embraces the wisdom that excellent health depends on a return to real foods and life-affirming practices. Her approach is not a quick-fix diet, but a step-by-step program to better understand the principles that lead to wholeness and health. If you would like to work with Camille to create your own vibrant health, contact her at camille@camillewatson.com.

Camille received her certification as a Health Coach from the Institute for Integrative Nutrition®. Her time at IIN® was instructive, healing and life-changing. If you would like to know more about IIN®, go to www.camillewatson.com and click on "Becoming a Health Coach."

Camille's pursuit of vibrant health extends beyond private consultations and the classroom to the hiking trails of the Great Smokey Mountains where she can be found many a weekend morning in the company of her very significant other, Brad.

Made in the USA
Middletown, DE
11 November 2017